PRAISE FOR

POSTPARTUM 30

"No matter how much planning you do, you can't control what happens when you give birth. But what the amazing Dr. Kristal Lau so brilliantly teaches, is that you can control what comes next. Having a medically trained professional who bridges modern and traditional health practices by your side, you'll be able to create a postpartum journey filled with bonding, serenity, and love. I only wish I'd had Kristal in my own early journey of motherhood."

—DR. ABBY MEDCALF, PhD, psychologist, author, TEDx speaker

"This book [is] ideal for expectant parents and their respective families with different cultures on how to manage postpartum. What I enjoyed was the inclusion of the male spouses and partners during this time, which, during traditional times, they were excluded. The author gives excellent explanations and modern medicine during the postpartum period and the changes between them with suggestions on how to manage this time. It has personal storie; recipes and menus; and support suggestions for the partner, spouse, Dad and family. It is easy to read and easy to make references whenever you would need to."

—DR. KAVIPRIYA SOMA, General practitioner obstetrician (GPO),
Athena Women's Clinic, Australia

"*Postpartum 30* is a thought-provoking and educational read for . . . mums-to-be who wish to find that perfect blend between traditional Chinese confinement practice and modern Western postpartum care in the fourth trimester. Kristal enthusiastically engages the reader in a conversational manner not unlike that used by an older sister or auntie. There is a deliberate absence of medical jargon in the text, and Kristal speaks to you through the pages deeply from her own upbringing and experiences. The text carefully simplifies difficult concepts of TCM and postpartum physiology to make them digestible to the layman mum, and the subsequent chapters are purposefully layered to incorporate these concepts—making them easy to recall on a practical level. The book also explores cultural nuances and social constructs of gender roles specific to the Malaysian-Chinese population. If you are looking for a guide on how to do confinement at home, this book is a great resource for the modern mum!"

—DR. GRACE CHAM, MBBS (Hons.), DRANZCOG,
Obstetrics and Gynaecology Trainee

"As a very western Caucasian growing up in Australia, I had never heard of a confinement month until I was pregnant with my first child. I was at work (as a GP) one day, and a patient who was also a white woman married to a Chinese Indonesian man asked me, 'So, has your mother-in-law planned your confinement yet?' You can probably imagine my response—a combination of 'what on earth are you talking about?' and 'I'm a grown woman, I plan my own things' especially when they relate to my body, my health, and now my children. Thankfully, no one expected me to last a month without washing!

"I do wish I'd had access to this book when I was pregnant. It would have helped me understand better some of the suggestions from my in-laws, and given me help finding that middle ground of respecting elders and their traditions whilst still acknowledging my own autonomy. Kristal does an excellent job of explaining traditional confinement practices in terms of social and cultural norms, and traditional Chinese medicine understandings. Then she takes this one step further and measures these up against modern lifestyle and modern Western medicine. The result is an easy read which ultimately gives the reader enough information to be able to pick and choose confinement practices that would suit them. I love how Kristal makes it clear that it doesn't have to be an all or nothing dichotomy—there really is scope to plan a confinement that truly suits your own circumstances. It would seem that the ultimate goal of even the most traditional confinement month is supporting the mother and ensuring her and her baby's health. With her own cultural experience and her medical knowledge, Kristal is able to distill down this goal in each aspect of the confinement, which is where she really gives you the power to decide what would be best for you. I can see this being of benefit to new Asian mothers around the globe, and to women like myself, partnered into the culture.

"As a General Practitioner with a special interest in perinatal care, I look forward to recommending this book to new mothers who are considering options for their confinement month."

—DR. SARAH TEDJASUKMANA, MBBS BSc (adv) (Hons I) DCH FRACGP, GP and co-founder of Sydney Perinatal Doctors

"I found [this to be] an extremely well-balanced book, encouraging solutions and suggestions for the relationship between traditional and modern medical practices postpartum. It encourages personal preferences for families with different cultures and gives ideas for problem solving in the postpartum period."

—SHAYNE WELLS, Retired Midwife

POSTPARTUM
30

POSTPARTUM
30

POSTPARTUM
30

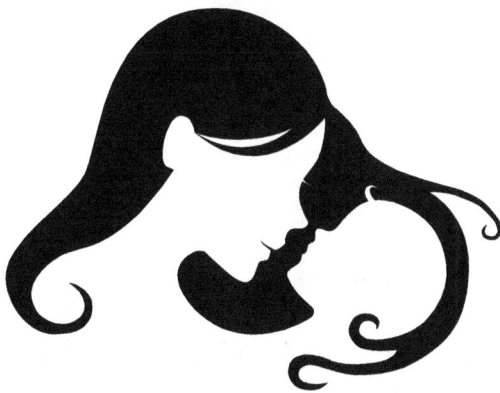

THIRTY DAYS TO A
NURTURED FOURTH TRIMESTER

KRISTAL LAU, MBBS

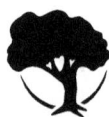

Published by

**MANDALA
TREE** PRESS
mandalatreepress.com

Paperback ISBN: 9781954801547
Hardcover with Dust Jacket ISBN: 9781954801578
Case Laminate Hardcover ISBN: 9781954801554
eBook ISBN: 9781954801561

HEA041000 HEALTH & FITNESS / Pregnancy & Childbirth
HEA024000 HEALTH & FITNESS / Women's Health
FAM032000 FAMILY & RELATIONSHIPS / Parenting / Motherhood

Cover design and typesetting by Kaitlin Barwick
Edited by Deborah Spencer and Lauren Woodbury

bridgesinhealth.com/postpartumbook
mamaswingwoman.com

For my mother, Josephine; my aunt Margaret;
and my late grandmother Yap Yoke Lan:
You represent the generation
of women before me.

For my girls, Kira and Kara:
The generation who will come after me.

And for my peers, today's generation of mothers:
I am you. You are me.
Sisters-in-arms, I look forward to taking
this journey of motherhood with you.

DISCLAIMER

This book contains recommendations and information relating to the postpartum period, matrescence, Malaysian Chinese postpartum cultural and traditional practices, basic Traditional Chinese Medicine (TCM) concepts, and trigger topics such as depression and suicidal thoughts.

The content in this book is not intended to substitute medical advice or to claim that one cultural practice is better than another. Please use this book as a supplement rather than replacement of regular advice and care of your health providers. This also applies to your racial, ethnic, and family cultures and traditions.

Every woman, female, and birthing person is different. Always seek professional medical advice from qualified health practitioners for any questions you may have about a medical or health condition, as well as treatments. Buying and reading this book does not establish a doctor-patient relationship between you, the reader, and the author, Kristal Lau.

Contents

Contents

Foreword

by Anne Yu Ming Gim

K ristal and I started with a therapeutic patient-pharmacist relationship. She was seeking *zuò yuè zi* (confinement) herbs to supplement and boost her recovery after giving birth while living here in Germany. "Wow, that's not a common request from my German patients!" I thought she was a German lady wanting to try the Chinese confinement practice. Receiving a request from a fellow Malaysian for confinement herbs was the last thing on my mind!

I head the Traditional Chinese Medicine (TCM) department of an apotheke south of Munich (*apotheke* means "pharmacy" in German). My speciality lies in bridging Western and Eastern medicine and herbal preparations for my patients. I take things a step further in my apotheke by offering my patients the option of purchasing pre-brewed herbs that are conserved to last for 6 months. We also offer granules of the herbs and we mix them according to the prescriptions.

Incorporating these modern techniques of herbal preparation has improved my patients' compliance in completing their herbal prescription course due to the convenience of consuming the herbs. This has made TCM more acceptable to the West because the herbs are presented in familiar Western dosage forms, and my German patients are comfortable with that. This is what I see in the future of health and wellness: the embracing of modernity and traditions. This book is a beautiful representation of this bridge between both worlds, especially in the realm of postpartum care and recovery. I think Kristal does a wonderful job of addressing this unique challenge of "modern versus tradition" in postpartum care. She gives the modern mom courage to put themselves first while maintaining a connection to their roots.

Anne Yu Ming Gim

BSc (Pharm) (Honours)
National University of Singapore
Deutsche Approbation als Apothekerin
Regierung von Oberbayern

Member of DECA (Germany)
"Gesellschaft für die Dokumentation von Erfahrungsmaterial der Chinesischen Arzneitherapie"
(translates as "Society for Documentation of Therapeutic Experiences with Chinese Medicine")

Preface

A Love Note for You, Dear Reader

Dear new moms, being pregnant can be rough. Or easy. Either way, you really don't have much control over how your pregnancy goes. Anything can happen anytime. No matter how much you prepare or "do things right." Same goes for your birth. Our birth plans are really just wishful thinking. Even for the "easiest" ones. Our body and baby will do whatever they want and need to.

Naturally, that means we've been out of control for pretty much the entire process of growing and birthing our babies. That can be difficult to accept. Jarring. Frustrating.

So when you're able to design and carry out a postpartum plan that focuses on your unique recovery and growth needs during the vulnerable time immediately after birth, how refreshing is that? You'll have a strong foundation to start your motherhood journey. And you can build upon this as you traverse the rest of the journey.

There's also something special about reconnecting with an ancient motherhood rite of passage. In our still very patriarchal society, there are still expectations that a modern mom should be able to do it all without a village or tribe to support them. The postpartum practice described in this book will give you space to be vulnerable and encourage others to help you without judgement. It's time to return to normalizing needing help and accepting help as mothers.

This book will show you that you deserve to have the support you need. And it is my wish that the information here will free you to ask for help without guilt and shame. We've got to nurture you so that you can grow into your new role and identity with all the love and respect you deserve.

WHO IS THIS BOOK FOR?

This book serves as a practical guide to plan and prepare for your postpartum recovery practice.

As a new mom, a postpartum plan is something you have some control over. Your pregnancy, birth, and new baby all have a mind of their own. Having this little bit of control is important if your birth plan didn't quite go according to plan (pun intended!). Or if your pregnancy was challenging, even if you were really fit and healthy to begin with. Your new baby? I wish you luck with anything going to plan. But at the very least, your chance of successfully following a postpartum recovery plan is a lot higher. This book can help you prepare for a postpartum recovery tailored to your liking.

If you're like me, an Asian woman who has migrated overseas, or you were born and grew up overseas, particularly in a Western country, this book is a wonderful resource on how to find and adjust what you need in order to design a postpartum recovery that resonates with you. I believe that you'll feel seen throughout this book. You'll feel relieved to know that you can adapt tradition and customs to your modern lifestyle and identity. And most important, you'll learn how to connect with the older generation while adapting a postpartum practise rooted in tradition. I see you, I hear you, I am you.

If you married into an Asian family, particularly an East Asian family (e.g. the Chinese, Japanese, Thais, Koreans, Indonesians, Filipinos, Taiwanese, and more), you'll find explanations on why your in-laws would want you to follow a specific postpartum recovery practice after having your child. In this case, the Chinese postpartum recovery practice of *zuò yuè zi* or confinement. You'll also find ways to compromise with them on some strict traditional practices so that you can have a postpartum recovery month suited to you.

Finally, if you're someone who wants to learn how to be a new mom's ally and postpartum support person (whether you're a new mom's spouse, partner, family member, or friend), this book will guide you on how to help your loved one carry out and complete their postpartum recovery practice in comfort and confidence. I promise you that the effort, space, and patience that you put into completing this postpartum recovery month will be treasured forever. It'll strengthen your bond, respect, and trust between each other.

So, don't wait too long to plan your postpartum recovery, especially if you're choosing to practice the recovery parts that require Chinese herbs and ingredients that aren't readily available in your area. Since we're also living in a time when disease outbreaks easily travel around the globe, having a postpartum plan beforehand helps steady your worries and anxieties about how to manage when you get home with a newborn.

A good time to start preparing is at the start of your third trimester of your pregnancy (around week 30) so that you're still able to travel if need be. If you want to include Traditional Chinese Medicine (TCM) in your postpartum recovery practice, this'll give you plenty of time to find and consult with a TCM doctor and get your herbs and food preparations ready. If you also need to plan things around your mother or mother-in-law, it's definitely a good time to do so before the baby is here. I'll guide you through this in chapter 3.

This book is split into two sections. Section one describes how to prepare for the physiological, emotional, and social changes you will go through during pregnancy and the postpartum period. Section two coaches you how to combine traditional and modern practices to create the perfect blend for your individual postpartum journey.

Terms & Definitions

I am a fan of defining words and terms whenever I write. This is a habit that I developed during my medical practice because I needed to be on the same wavelength as my patients, their families, and my colleagues. Carrying this habit into this book helps keep you, my dear reader, and me on the same page (pun intended!) and allows us to speak the same language as you read this book.

When the terms **health practitioners** and **health providers** are used in this book, they include doctors, nurses, nurse practitioners, midwives, therapists/counsellors, TCM doctors/practitioners, allied health professionals, doulas, and pharmacists. Not all women have access to doctors. Many times, nurses, midwives, and doulas play a large role in managing the postpartum period.

New Mom(s) in this book refers to women and female readers who identify as mothers and are first-time mothers or are having more children. Every pregnancy and childbirth experience is unique. And we're always a "new mom of (insert new number of children)." Thus, those of you who have a newborn, no matter how many times before, are referred to as a new mother in this book.

Postpartum Period is when the body takes 6 to 8 weeks to return to its pre-pregnancy state. This begins immediately after the delivery of the placenta.

The Postpartum Year is my take on the clinical definition of the postpartum period above. I define it as up to 1 year for some of us to return to the pre-pregnancy state; physically (our body's outside), physiologically (our body's insides), mentally, and emotionally.

Fourth Trimester is the first 3 months after giving birth.

Modern Confinement is the 30 days of postpartum recovery at home after giving birth. Related to the traditional Chinese postpartum practice of *zuò yuè zi* (a.k.a., "sitting the month").

Introduction

Making the Case for a Modern Confinement

Were you brought up in Asia or in the West by Asian parents with conflicting messages about sticking to traditional values but to also embracing modernity to avoid being left behind in the modern rat race?

"I'm giving you all this education so that you can provide for yourself in the future. Also, when will you be getting married? You're in your mid-twenties and still single! You need a husband to look after you."

Or perhaps you've got Asian in-laws who are pretty conservative?

"Yes, lah, I understand she's Westernised. Very independent. But she's now your wife, she has to follow you, lah! Have to follow our family's traditions, mah."

The confusion and conflict can easily extend into your pregnancy and postpartum experience.

Why? Asian women, in general, practice a period of confinement or "sitting in" after giving birth. So, without saying so, the female elders in your family will expect you to follow this tradition after giving birth. They'll happily show up to help you through this time along with their motherly advice: solicited and unsolicited ones!

Each Asian culture and family have their version of this postpartum practice. This book is dedicated to the Chinese confinement practice, a reflection of my Malaysian-Chinese heritage.

WHAT IS THE CONFINEMENT PRACTICE?

This Chinese postpartum practice is known as 坐月子 (zuò yuè zi), "sitting the month," "doing the month," or confinement, because the new mom, and their newborn, are confined to their home. This practice is a postpartum recovery program meant to help new moms regain energy and strength for the motherhood and parenthood journey ahead. It is also believed that adhering to the various confinement rules can prevent future ailments, such as rheumatism, when a mother reaches old age. These rules are formed from Traditional Chinese Medicine (TCM) principles. We explore more of this in chapter 1.

While I knew I was going to follow the confinement practice after giving birth, I didn't like how constricting some of the rules and practices were. Viewing them through the lens of my medical training and experience, I felt that some of these rules and practices wouldn't help me get and stay comfortable while I recovered from birth. Some of them can be a health risk too!

"Don't wash your hair or take a shower for 30 days after you give birth, ya!"

"And you have to stay warm and eat and drink warm food and beverages all the time. If you don't, the wind will go into your body. That'll make you get all sorts of aches and pain when you're old!"

*"Most importantly, don't **layan**[1] any strong feelings during these 30 days, ya? Not good for you and baby. Just focus on the good and happy things!"*

From a personal perspective, I felt these rules hadn't changed much from my mom's and grandmother's time. They seemed out of touch with how I viewed myself as a mixed modern-traditional woman.

I was born and brought up in Kuala Lumpur, Malaysia. As a 1990s kid, my teenage years were filled with Western pop culture from MTV, Hollywood films, and TV series like *Xena the Warrior Princess*, *Angel*, and *Charmed*. The Western export of being a woman who could hold her own, fight her own battles, and thrive without a man was pretty inspiring. My mom didn't mind me watching those shows either. She raised me to be independent after all.

I also had equal exposure to Chinese culture and shows since my parents and grandparents followed Hong Kong movies and TV series religiously through a Malaysian cable service called Astro. (Fellow Malaysians, remember the *Wah Lai Toi* channel with all the Hong Kong TV series? *Journey to the West* and *A Kindred Spirit*?) Many female characters were portrayed as docile, gentle, and almost fairy-like. Those who could fight were the "troublesome" characters (like Fong Sai

---

1. *layan*: Malay word for "entertain" or "give in."

3

Yuk's mother in the Hong Kong TVB series). I saw myself in those rebellious female characters. I admired them.

I also grew up following Malaysian cultural traditions, specifically Chinese traditions and taboos, since my ancestors are from South China. I'm a third generation Malaysian, so many Chinese customs from mainland China have been adapted to Malaysia's multicultural melting pot.

Once such custom relates to the Hungry Ghost month. This time is usually observed in August, which corresponds to the seventh month in the lunar calendar. And what a time of trepidation! I was always told to watch my back for wandering souls from hell who were visiting the mortal realm. And to avoid stepping on any offerings that littered the sidewalk or were placed under many big trees.

Pregnant women were especially cautioned against going out alone at night during this month. Well, they weren't supposed go out at night at all! The spirits might've taken advantage of the vulnerable state of the pregnant person. And if they could help it, they SHOULD NOT give birth during this month. This belief is followed up till today for some folks.

I'm also a solid follower of *feng shui* because my mom still practices it diligently. So, to not adhere to the customs and taboos I grew up with made me feel very uncomfortable. Despite being a woman of science!

Naturally, I had a period of confusion and conflict about whether I had to be modern or conservative. But during my years as a medical doctor, I became comfortable with my modern and traditional identities. I embraced both sides of myself.

It started with patients and their families asking shyly,

"Kristal, erm, is it okay if we wanted to try acupuncture to try to improve Dad's feeling in his arms? The stroke rehabilitation doesn't seem to be working yet."

"Doc, I don't really want to take medications for this cold. Can I have some herbal teas I used to drink as a kid?"

"I'm a bit embarrassed to ask but I want to try Reiki healing for my back pain. What do you think?"

My response? Yes, yes, and yes! The catch? As long as the complementary therapies and herbal concoctions don't interfere or worsen the main problem. I always found their expression of relief to my answer intriguing. Because in my mind, "Why wouldn't you try both? It's so normal in Malaysia to use both traditional medicine and modern medicine."

This frequent exchange made me realise, "I CAN be a woman of science and follow traditional practices if I wish!" There was such a relief in releasing myself from the belief that I had to choose one side or the other.

After a while of having these interactions, I realised that embracing this side of me gave me an edge to my clinical practice. I could easily build a connection with my patients and their families or caregivers because of my mixed modern-traditional upbringing and approach. This has given me the open-mindedness and humility in letting my patients guide me in how best to serve them.

It is this part of me that is imbued in this book. The part of me that always seeks to compromise so that I can preserve tradition and be true to myself.

So while I planned for my confinement month while pregnant with each of my children, I wanted to have an experience that complemented my mixed modern-traditional self. A confinement version that relates to our modern life yet rooted in my heritage.

I knew that if I was made to follow the traditional confinement rules strictly, there was a high chance I wouldn't complete the postpartum practice as desired. And I'd feel uncomfortable and stressed rather than pampered and rested!

Here lies the challenge with asking the modern generation to strictly follow traditional rules. Why?

CHALLENGES OF A TRADITIONAL CONFINEMENT

Outdated to the Modern Woman

Every generation always wants the next to do better. Many women in the past had to endure so much humiliation, degradation, and barriers to education and basic human rights. We definitely don't want this to continue for us and the future generation! Yet, there are still degrees of humiliation, degradation, and barriers to education and basic human rights for women in our twenty-first century. Just pop on the news and there's plenty to read about gender inequities globally across all aspects of human life.

The modern woman has unique challenges compared to the older generation of women. We bear the burden of breaking the cycle of oppression and sacrifice our maternal elders had to make through no complete fault of their own. We also bear the burden of setting examples for our children to show them that it is possible to break the cycle and do better.

Modern women everywhere these days also have to think about how much maternity leave they and their partner or spouse can get. Is it financially and logistically feasible to carry out a very traditional confinement month? Can they get the physical support to do it? There were less of these challenges back in the days when families lived with each other in the same village or neighbourhood. We once knew our neighbours really well and trusted many of them. This connection isn't as common nowadays.

Excludes Partners from the Postpartum Period

Historically, males and fathers weren't allowed into the birthing room or during confinement. It was considered bad luck for fathers to come into contact with the birthing process. Meaning, bad luck would befall the family from then on if he did! (See the upcoming excerpt on "A Note on Chinese Cultural Views and Traditions Related to Postpartum and the Female Body" for more explanation.)

Some folks still believe in this taboo today! Others just stick to tradition and don't question it regardless of whether they agree with that belief. Many men, males, fathers, and dads end up being excluded from the confinement month. This means they're missing out on bonding time with their newborns. And they're unable to learn early on how to care for their loved one and baby for the rest of the Postpartum Year. This exclusion still happens in some confinement centers in East Asia.

The problem with this exclusion is just that. Benched. "Get out of the way!" is the message. Worst of all is the insinuation that "you don't know how to be a parent." But women are not born "knowing" how to parent just like that. We're not in the Matrix where the arrival of a baby can be programmed to automatically upload a "parenting manual." So, how are men and fathers expected to know how to parent if they don't learn hands on?

> *Note:* I challenge this exclusion head on throughout the book with a focus in chapter 8 to ensure men and fathers are included in the confinement month. I'll say it now to plant the idea: *Spouses, partners, men, and fathers should be the PRIMARY postpartum recovery support person!*

Inconvenient in Our Modern World

Folks of Chinese ethnicity live all over the world nowadays. Many migrate to Western countries. Sure, Chinatowns are set up in most major Western cities, but not everything one needs for the confinement month is always available there. For those of us living in areas without access to Chinese herbs and special ingredients for cooking and making confinement meals and beverages, having to follow a strict tradition means we probably can't practice it much at all!

We've also got great health services and amenities in many Western and developing countries. Sanitation isn't like in the olden days anymore. We've got water treatment facilities and waste processing plants. We've got heating and cooling technologies that grow more advanced as time goes by. Most of all, we've got modern medicine and preventive programs to manage diseases that used to be fatal back in the days. So, strict traditions around hygiene are becoming more of an inconvenience in our modern world.

The biggest problem with being strict with old traditions is the loss of tradition itself. When we don't continue observing tradition in our generation, it's easy to see how it will be forgotten by the next generation. And just because something is outdated, doesn't mean we should discard it. When there's room for adaptation, growth, and all parties can come together to preserve a tradition, we've got to seize the moment!

A NOTE ON CHINESE CULTURAL VIEWS AND TRADITIONS

Way back in ancient Chinese times, as described in *The Book of Rites*,[2] a new mom and her newborn were isolated after birth for 3 months. This is because it was believed that it was unlucky for the father and other family members to come into contact with the birthing process. This is undoubtedly the early version of the confinement practice.

It's also very common among many Asian cultures to view a woman's blood as "dirty." Back in Malaysia, I've been told that some places of worship don't allow entry to women who are having their menses. Because that blood is "dirty," it's "bad luck" and "offensive" to have her in a place of worship at that time. I've also heard of very traditional families who would "hide" the girl or woman away until her menses cycle ended. This relates to the view that childbirth is a "dirty" process.

> *"The reason for a woman to fulfil the month after childbirth is because during the birth her body passes through a state of pollution. Before her lochia is cleansed, she is not allowed to go outdoors, neither to approach the locations of wells and stoves, nor to worship the spirits and attend ancestral sacrifices."*
>
> —Xiao Pin Fang[3]

Keep in mind that TCM and Chinese culture are closely intertwined. So, there are traditions and practices that can be both medicinal and cultural.

---

2. "The Book of Rites, The Birth of a Child," World History Commons, https://world historycommons.org/book-rites-birth-child.
3. Jen-Der Lee, "Childbirth in Early Imperial China," *NAN NÜ* volume 7, Issue 2 (2005), https://doi.org/10.1163/156852605775248658.

Keeping to the very traditional and strict practices of confinement is a disservice to modern moms and their families. Being rigid with tradition, when our modern world isn't designed to support modern moms and their families, risks worsening the health of new moms. Then the tradition itself risks being forgotten.

If the postpartum confinement recovery practice continues to be outdated, it's going to be perceived as more inconvenient and uncomfortable for new moms and their families to follow. It's no wonder if the younger generation would rather dismiss the practice than try it out.

Yet, there is merit in preserving this practice. How so?

BENEFITS OF A TRADITIONAL CONFINEMENT

Remembering Our Roots

While traditions can be preserved in writing, audio, and visual form, there's something magical about experiencing it ourselves. The memories we form when we engage all or some of our five senses are unparalleled. I've noticed that many skills and practices are usually passed down by "see one, do one, teach one."[4] Our ancestors who didn't have access to education

---

4. In medicine, I was taught many ward-based clinical procedural skills this way (i.e., not complex procedures requiring the operating theatre). I learned by watching tutorials or observing someone else perform the procedure. Or by attending a simulation session. Then, I'd do one under supervision. And when a junior or medical student wanted to learn the procedure, I'd be the one to teach them. My clinical educators emphasized that this was a practical way to keep our skills sharp and up-to-date. I follow this guide today in most things I do. This method of learning also happens at home. Especially with food and crafts. We're always learning from our elders about family recipes, tips, and tricks in the kitchen (and in their art and craft). Then, we practice it till we get better. And then we teach it to our children!

or were illiterate have been passing down their stories, culture, and traditions this way!

The best method of remembering the ways of confinement is to experience it ourselves. Knowing what worked and didn't work for us is a valuable resource for planning our next confinement after the next child. We're also able to help others who are looking for tips and tricks before and during their confinement month.

Passing Down Our Heritage

We know the power of stories. Storytelling has been around since the time of cavemen and ancient civilisations. Knowledge, religion, and traditions have been passed down this way. Nations have been moved, rallied, and crumbled through stories. Combined with our memories of our confinement month, being able to tell our story of experiencing this rite of motherhood and parenthood is an unforgettable way of passing down a part of our heritage. What a wonderful way of sharing your journey into and through motherhood and parenthood with your children too!

If you and your spouse or partner are the first to raise a mixed-race family, this holds even more value because you're both able to pass down your joint heritage once you've tailored a confinement practice to your family.

Honouring Our Elders

Coming together with our elders to nurture the new mom is becoming more difficult now than before. Sure, we have modern travel methods compared to our ancestors but we're also more dispersed around the world. Many of us adult children are also modern immigrants to Western countries or to another place that our parents feel holds a better future for us and our kids. It also isn't always affordable for our parents to fly overseas or their health can't tolerate the ever-narrowing flight seats on long-haul journeys.

Continuing to practice confinement offers us a chance to reconnect with our elders when we're planning for the postpartum recovery month. It's a wonderful time to come together and rediscover family traditions and family histories. Especially as a way to take a walk in the shoes of the women who came before us. I can only imagine the new or stronger bonds a modern mom will form with their mothers, aunts, stepmoms, grandmothers—well, all the mom figures in their lives! I'd imagine not many elders openly share their stories of triumph and failures when they first became a mother. I cannot think of a better way to honour our matriarch elders than to hold space for them and remind them that they're not invisible.

This is also a perfect opportunity to have open conversations about what you, the modern mom, needs. It's such a tender conversation, so I'd like to think that our elders would be more empathetic to the new challenges the modern world brings to new moms and their families.

This book exists because I wanted to share my experience and remember the history of Chinese postpartum confinement in English. Something I can pass down to my children so that they and their partners can easily follow this tradition should they choose to.

I am not fluent or literate in Mandarin, Cantonese, or any other Chinese dialects. I can only speak enough to order delicious food at the stalls and curse at someone. And I'm not sure if my children will pick up the language since they're unlikely to grow up and live around Mandarin- and Chinese-dialect-speaking family and communities.

I also don't like being shamed for not being able to speak my mother tongue or pressured into learning the language when it's not my priority. So, I wanted to share a resource with those of you who don't know Mandarin or are unlikely to pick up the language anytime soon. Just like me!

Making the conscious effort to respectfully adapt and adjust an old practice to our modern world means putting in effort to build a bridge (or many bridges!) between modernity and tradition. Between mothers and adult daughters. Between generations. Across cultures in mixed marriages.

And there is no right or wrong way to do it.

This book describes my method of adapting the traditional confinement practice to our modern needs and lifestyle. My recommendations come from bridging my medical background with my Malaysian upbringing, which was heavily influenced by TCM. My mom and aunt were also consulted, as well as a TCM practitioner, Dr. Eun Kim, who practices in Los Angeles, United States.

This book also serves as your guide and life jacket for the mental and emotional whirlpool that is the Postpartum Year. The postpartum recovery period is a very vulnerable time for new moms, no matter how many kids you've had. This is because it's always a new life event that's happening. There's so much physical, emotional, and mental recovery to go through plus the constant self-growth as your identity as a new mom and parent, and as a modern woman and person, is challenged every step of the way.

So, I invite you to embrace this month of being nurtured in the first 30 days of your postpartum recovery period. Allow me and your support network to help you get comfortable at the beginning of your postpartum journey.

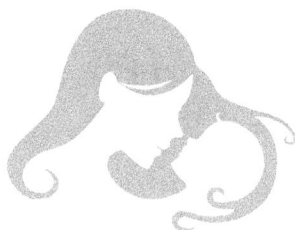

Section 1

The Postpartum Journey

Chapter 1

Postpartum Physiology

This isn't a medical textbook, so why is there a chapter on physiology? Because we don't celebrate enough about how amazing our bodies are even after pregnancy and giving birth! To grow life for up to 9 months and then endure marathon-level exertion to give birth is one thing. To then be tasked overnight with keeping a precious baby alive while our body immediately gets to work on returning to its pre-pregnancy state is mind blowing.

There's no rest, is there?

Yet, we do it. YOU, dear new mom, do it anyway!

This knowledge of postpartum physiology helps us start forgiving ourselves for our flawed moments during our recovery period. And for the rest of the Postpartum Year.

I promise you'll be even more amazed at yourself after reading this chapter.

First, some terms and definitions to introduce.

POSTPARTUM PERIOD DEFINED

Postpartum literally means "after childbirth."[5] But we don't say that a new mom is in postpartum forever. There's a time frame associated with postpartum.

Why Is It Important to Define the Postpartum Time Frame?

First, the physiological changes after giving birth—the changes inside your body—take about 6 to 8 weeks to return to the pre-pregnancy state. This includes hormonal changes, the uterus shrinking, and the abdominal contents "re-shuffling" once a baby has vacated the womb. This time is also called the puerperium. If things don't resolve by this time frame, it's important to get checked out and have any health conditions diagnosed and treated on time. We'll delve more into this in the section below "Postpartum Physiology—The Basics."

Second, having a time frame allows health providers, businesses, and educators to focus on problems that are unique to the postpartum period. Examples of postpartum problems and conditions include postpartum depression, diastasis recti, and a weak pelvic floor. The time frame also gives care providers direction in curating specialised care plans, products, and services, and to better monitor your postpartum health. For example, baby blues and postpartum depression are different in the timing of when they usually start and how long they last. Understanding this is crucial in knowing how to support you through the baby blues and to keep an eye out for postpartum depression.

---

5. *Merriam-Webster.com Dictionary*, s.v. "postpartum," accessed July 18, 2022, https://www.merriam-webster.com/dictionary/postpartum.

Finally, giving the postpartum period a time frame allows health providers to transfer care if that's required. It also gives the next health provider a guide on where to pick up from. For example, the OBGYN specialist usually has an official follow-up with new moms at 6 weeks postpartum. If all is well after that appointment, they'll usually transfer care to a family doctor, nurse practitioner (NP), or general practitioner (GP). So, if a new mom was diagnosed with postpartum depression and started treatment under the OBGYN's care during the 6 weeks after birth, they will likely continue their care plan with a GP or NP after that.

However, note that nuances exist in every country because it's important for medical guidelines to cater to women in that country. So, dear readers, if there's variation in how postpartum care is carried out in your country, it's likely due to the current standard guidelines of the OBGYN association in your country.

So, What Is the Current Definition of Postpartum Period?

The starting point of the postpartum period is very clear. It begins immediately after babies are born. Clinically, it begins immediately after the birth of the placenta. But the end point of this period isn't as clear. Currently, science and medicine has found that it generally takes 6 to 8 weeks after giving birth for the recovery of the many organs and internal systems involved (skin included!). So, modern healthcare professionals worldwide use this time frame now.

However, there's more recognition that the postpartum period can be up to 12 weeks after delivery (hence the term,

Fourth Trimester) and even up to a year.[6] This is an evolving space. So, there's a chance that this time frame will change in the future when there's more data to advocate for that.

Why Do Health Definitions Evolve?

Science and modern medicine are not always set in stone. This is because scientific and medical communities learn new things about the human body every day. Same goes for traditional medicine. So, guidelines are always updated to reflect our population's current needs and knowledge. This flexibility is very important so that health professionals can provide the best care based on what they know right now.

With regards to the postpartum period, there's a lot to learn (and unlearn!) about what a new mom needs for their recovery. Sure, there's a lot of clinical knowledge about what the body does after birth to get back to pre-pregnancy condition. But health programs, policies, and laws (and our society's mindset) don't always keep up with what the modern mom truly needs for their postpartum health.

Good health is so much more than just the absence of disease. Your social and emotional well-being, and your mental health, are also part of your postpartum health. So, streamlined postpartum care must evolve to more personalised care based on where you live, the resources and social support available to you, your socioeconomic status, your culture, and your identity.

6. Pamela Berens, *Overview of the postpartum period: Normal physiology and routine maternal care*, Charles J Lockwood (Wolters Kluwer UpToDate, 2021), https://www-uptodate-com.ezproxy3.lhl.uab.edu/contents/overview-of.

I follow the definition of health as per WHO: *"Health is a state of complete physical, mental and social well-being and not merely the absence of disease or infirmity."*[7] So, by this definition, I'd hazard a guess that many of us new moms DON'T HAVE GOOD HEALTH. Because while our physical body will have recovered to some extent during the 6-8 weeks after birth, our mental and social well-being still requires attention for longer than that.

For this shift in postpartum care to happen (and to support those who are already shifting to personalised postpartum care models), the postpartum period definition must be able to evolve too!

So, I'm very glad that the modern physicians in obstetrics are very open to redefining the postpartum period as "12 weeks after birth" or even "up to 1 year after birth." This shows that they're in touch about what the modern mom needs and wants today. Not tomorrow, not yesterday—TODAY.

And that's just in line with what motherhood and parenthood is in the early years, isn't it? Just doing what we can for what we, our kids, and our families need TODAY.

Right now, we modern moms need postpartum care for a lot longer than just 6–8 weeks after birth.

In this book, I'll be using the definition of the postpartum period as "up to 1 year after giving birth." I call this "The Postpartum Year." Meaning, it takes up to 1 year for some of us to return to the pre-pregnancy state; physically (our body's outside), physiologically (our body's insides), mentally, and emotionally.

I'll be using the term "Postpartum Year" from here onward.

---

7. "Constitution of the World Health Organization," World Health Organization, https://www.who.int/about/governance/constitution.

A BLAST TO THE PAST: MATERNAL AND INFANT SURVIVAL PRE-MODERN ERA

Infant and maternal mortality rates were scarily high back in the olden days. This meant that many new moms and newborns didn't survive. Sure, certain conditions like the breech foetal position and foetal shoulder dystocia were known about back then and had treatment plans in place. But the risk of disability or poor health after the procedure were high for moms and the newborn due to the overall rudimentary medical technology and knowledge.

Then there's the more complicated pregnancy or birth-related conditions such as HELLP syndrome (a life-threatening condition affecting the blood and liver through Hemolysis, Elevated Liver enzymes, and Low Platelet count), which was generalised as convulsions or sickness. Many mothers and newborns did not survive such conditions.

Poor sanitation and primitive infrastructure in the ancient era, such as wood-heating furnaces and stoves, also contributed to poor maternal and infant health. Overall, it's easy to see that pregnancy and childbirth were (and still are for some populations) incredibly dangerous, life-threatening events.

Another example, we know today that Vitamin K is essential for blood clotting. But in newborns, their immature gut is unable to make Vitamin K efficiently. Vitamin K also doesn't cross the placenta easily and so, it is not transferred in great amounts via the breastmilk. So, before vitamin K injections became available, many newborns were at high-risk of bleeding in the brain, leading to disability or death.

Therefore, for a mother and newborn to survive the birthing process pre-modern era, that was pretty miraculous! For both to make it to one month, that was a very good sign that mom and baby should continue to thrive.[8]

---

8. "Chinese Birth Rituals," Singapore Infopedia, last modified 14 May 2013, https://eresources.nlb.gov.sg/infopedia/articles/SIP_2013-05-14_113920.html.

PHYSIOLOGICAL CHANGES POSTPARTUM

To make a bunch of health information easier to digest, I'm paraphrasing a clinical resource about these changes according to the systems and organs of our body.[9] It's easier to visualise these changes one body part at a time.

I don't expect you to memorise or remember any of this. I definitely don't want to scare or overwhelm you as you read this section. I'm writing this to inform you about the good, bad, beautiful, and ugly that can happen during the Postpartum Year. When you have such information, there are four things you'll gain:

1. More confidence to ask questions about your concerns and curiosities while you recover after birth. There's no such thing as stupid questions!

2. A newfound respect for your body. This is very helpful for when you're ready to reframe how you view your postpartum body and self. It also helps with adjusting our expectations in how we tackle our transition into motherhood.

3. Solidarity that you're not alone in all the chaos that is postpartum. Postpartum recovery takes time. You need time to regain energy and strengthen your health. So, you can and should ask for help when you need to! We have to stop peddling the rhetoric of the Super-Modern-Mom-Parent-Do-It-All-Superhero which can damage both moms' and their families' health.

---

9. See Pamela Berens, *Overview of the postpartum period: Normal physiology and routine maternal care*, Charles J Lockwood (Wolters Kluwer UpToDate, 2021), https://www.uptodate-com.ezproxy3.lhl.uab.edu/contents/overview-of; Giovanni Maciocia, *The Foundations of Chinese Medicine: A Comprehensive Text* (Elsevier, 2015).

4. Validation that the postpartum journey is difficult and challenging! I hope you'll start giving yourself permission to be kind and forgive yourself often in your postpartum journey. This time can be filled with wonderful moments and opportunities to grow as a person once you embrace this chaos.

POSTPARTUM EFFECTS ON SYSTEMS AND ORGANS

So much happens as soon as your baby is born!

You might get hit with the shivers within 1 to 30 minutes after giving birth. This could be due to many reasons; your body's response to its temperature falling after labour, bleeding, the placental separation, or the medications you've been given (if any).

You'll definitely be exhausted beyond belief after giving birth. But will you sleep immediately? Unlikely, since your hormones will be starting their roller-coaster cycles right after you deliver the placenta. The adrenaline rush from such an exciting yet traumatic and raw few hours will likely keep you awake for a while. Not to mention the health providers who'll visit your bedside often to check on you!

Sleep

Now, will you get more rest a week in? You'd be lucky to! There's a high chance of experiencing fatigue from sleep deprivation. This can easily happen because as a new mom, you'll likely be the primary carer of your newborn around the clock. You'll also likely be hyperaware of every little sound and movement your baby makes or doesn't make!

"Gosh, are they still breathing?" *stares at the baby in the crib or bassinet every 5 minutes to observe the rise and fall of their tiny chest*

*"Jeez! Why are they grunting so much in their sleep? Are they choking on their saliva? Or *gasp* are they choking on their spit up?"* *jumps to look at the baby in the crib or bassinet with every grunt they make*

"It's been 3 hours! Should I wake my baby? Or let them sleep?" *stares at the baby while making a decision*

Plus if you're nursing, it takes a lot of energy to produce breastmilk. When your little one is so new to life, they will be suckling for dear life (also known as cluster feeding) because the breast needs this cue to produce milk. This can mean nursing every 2 hours around the clock until your milk comes in, usually up to 5 days postpartum (this can vary for different women).

CHECK-IN TIME: HEY, YOU OKAY?

Questions? You probably have TONS of them. Write all of them down because that foggy mom brain is running so fast on so little energy, you might forget your questions.

Ask, ask, ask. Again and again. Your roller coaster hormones, sleep deprivation, and exhaustion can come together to create storms of anxiety and worry. If asking questions helps, do it. Need to hear the same answers again because it helps you feel better? Then ask again!

Here's a fact for you: You're providing your baby so much attention and you've been successful at keeping your newborn alive every day since giving birth. You also did that OVERNIGHT. Literally right after giving birth. AND THAT'S AMAZING!

If you're feeling overwhelmed, say this with me: *"I have just done the most amazing thing. I brought my baby into this world! And I'm feeding my baby the best I can. I'm tired and I'm hurting. And that's okay. It's hard and rough. And I can't get enough sleep. That's okay too. This will pass. We're new in this together too, baby. Let's try again tomorrow, together!"*

Weight

The average weight loss from delivering our baby and placenta, including the water breaking, is about 6 kg (13 lb.). This weight differs for each of us depending on the weight of our babies. No wonder I felt such an odd sense of hollowness in my belly right after my baby was born. I was sure my abdominal organs had no idea what to do with all that space after being squished for about 9 months!

You can easily lose another 2 to 7 kg (5 to 15 lb.) throughout the 6 to 8 weeks after giving birth. This comes from the ongoing contraction of the uterus, lochia loss, and losing the rest of the water retention accumulated during pregnancy.

To Weigh or Not to Weigh?

I can understand why you'd prefer not to weigh yourself in the Postpartum Year. After all, we've got enough societal pressure and sometimes family pressure around "bouncing back" as soon as possible after giving birth. You really don't need the scale to remind you of how much has changed in your weight and size during pregnancy!

In my family, and from what I've heard from my fellow Malaysian friends, there's this obsession about weight and size by the womenfolk.

"Aiyoh, you put on so much weight already! Why ah?"

"Girl, you better watch what you eat. Cannot be so big sized."

These comments are hurtful and insensitive. I mean, c'mon! I just had a baby within a year! I also don't want to go around advertising health issues or lifestyle and relationship stressors that may have affected my weight, such as my postpartum depression and solo-parenting my girls while my husband is deployed or constantly away for work.

Yet, we're told, "I'm just saying only!" when we mention that it's unkind to make such comments. This is a very Malaysian way of meaning, "I'm just making a comment. You don't have to listen to it." Our elders are used to their comments "going in one ear and out the other ear" if it's unwelcomed by the person they're speaking to. Unfortunately, the damage to our self-esteem and our emotional and mental health is done.

What ever happened to not saying anything if you've got nothing nice to say?

Yet, keeping track of your weight as you recover from birth is very important. Weight during pregnancy and in the 6 to 8 weeks after giving birth isn't just about muscles and fats. It includes how much water you're retaining or losing due to hormonal changes.

Some life-threatening conditions can show up early as water retention and rapid weight gain, such as kidney failure, liver failure, and heart failure. Knowing that your weight gain seems off for what you're expecting or what you're used to can help you advocate for your health. It's always better to catch an ailment earlier rather than later!

The takeaway point here is to watch for patterns in your weight change. The Postpartum Year brings many fluctuations to your body so it's more useful to you and your health provider to watch for and discuss patterns rather than raw number points.

Vital Signs

As the term itself says, these signs are important indicators of life!

Blood Pressure

Within the 24 hours of delivering the placenta, your blood pressure can be higher than your usual readings due to pain and/or excitement during labour and after birth. But normally, it should stay within your usual range throughout.

High blood pressure after birth that doesn't settle back to your usual range is a risk for postpartum pre-eclampsia and eclampsia (seizures and multi-organ dysfunction), similar to high blood pressure during pregnancy. Some of us may experience low blood pressure and that can be due to postpartum haemorrhage (extreme blood loss). This is why your health providers are so interested in checking your blood pressure often during and after the birth!

Body Temperature

Slight increase in body temperature can be from shivering and sweating, and/or the after-effects of the muscle contractions during labour and birth. The body temperature should return to normal (usually around 36.4°C to 37.2°C or 97.5°F to 98.9°F) within 12 hours of giving birth.

Something to be aware of: Fevers that come up on day 3 postpartum or later can indicate a brewing infection in the body. A temperature of 38°C (100.4°F) or higher is considered a fever. Take your temperature if you think you're feeling ill or having feverish symptoms like chills and shivers when your environment isn't cold. This vital sign is easy to keep an eye on at home with a digital thermometer.

Hormones

Our body's hormone system can be complex to understand even in the pre-pregnancy state. There are many feedback loops that constantly tell different organs what hormones to activate or pause depending on what we're eating, doing, and feeling. Now, add pregnancy, labour, and childbirth on top of that! The extra work and balancing our body has to do and adjust for the health of our growing baby and our pregnant self is highly demanding.

And the work doesn't stop there after you've given birth! Our body adjusts once again to return some parts to the pre-pregnancy state while other parts transform to prepare us to nourish and care for our newborn.

Note: Even medical professionals and scientists need time to understand our hormone systems so I definitely will not attempt to deliver anything remotely complex in this section. All you need to know are the basics of what type of hormones the postpartum body has to deal with and how that can affect you.

Oestrogen and Progesterone

These hormones usually drop drastically and suddenly after you give birth. Their functions are more important during pregnancy so once you've delivered your baby and placenta, it's time for them to dial things down. This sudden shift in oestrogen and progesterone levels will take time to stabilise. Unfortunately, during this time, you're likely at the mercy of the swinging moods that come with this hormonal imbalance. While this roller-coaster of emotions is common and temporary, it's still important to acknowledge and talk about anything you want to during this time.

Oxytocin

This hormone helps the uterus contract after giving birth. And it works with prolactin (below) to promote breastfeeding and mom-baby attachment after birth. It's also a stress-reducing hormone that helps reduce feelings of fear. The wonderful thing about oxytocin is that it has a positive feedback on itself. This means that once your pituitary gland releases oxytocin, the hormone will tell the gland to release more of it! This continues in the 6 to 8 weeks after giving birth.

Prolactin

The main hormone that stimulates breastmilk production. This is why if you choose to breastfeed and pump, you're usually taught to let your baby nurse on demand or pump regularly in the beginning. These actions tell the brain to release more prolactin to make more breastmilk. So, as long as there's demand (suckling and pumping), your body will keep producing prolactin to make breastmilk!

Endorphins

Our happy hormones that also help relieve pain! This is why some new moms have that warm and fuzzy feeling of joyful giddiness after giving birth and while breastfeeding. This helps new moms want to keep nursing because you're literally being rewarded with an emotional high whenever you do. And I say some of us feel that because there's also some of us who don't have that happy high (see the section about dysphoric milk ejection reflex; D-MER in chapter 2: The Postpartum Journey). These happy hormones can also be triggered when we're performing any caring activities for our newborn. There's no doubt that mothers are absolutely designed to be obsessed with the little ones!

Stress Hormones

Usually, these tend to drop after giving birth. The skin-to-skin time between new moms and newborns can further help decrease these stress hormones in both mom and baby. Unfortunately, our modern life and world can keep our stress levels and hormones up. Even more so if you've had a difficult pregnancy, labour, or needed a C-section. In the postpartum recovery time and the Postpartum Year, lack of emotional support and attention can be a risk for stress level and hormones to remain high.

Skin and Hair

Stretch marks will fade from red to silverish in colour, but they're permanent. The "mom pouch" or "mom belly"—that loose abdominal skin that can make you look pregnant months after delivery—may remain if the elastic skin fibres over that area tore during the pregnancy. Diastasis recti may also contribute to the ongoing "mom pouch" or "mom belly" loose skin if not corrected. See section "Abdominal Muscles" below for more about diastasis recti.

The patches of pigmentation of skin during pregnancy (chloasma) on the face, armpits, abdomen, and other sun-exposed areas will resolve over time.

Postpartum hair loss commonly happens 1 to 5 months after giving birth and usually returns to normal hair growth and loss pattern around 6 to 15 months after delivery. This hair-loss is accelerated from your usual hair-loss pattern due to the drop of oestrogen after giving birth. Therefore, there's a general recommendation by health providers to continue taking your prenatal vitamins in the Postpartum Year to help replenish the nutrients your body needs for recovery.

Breasts

There can be breast engorgement by the end of the first 24 hours after birth. This can be painful. The engorgement is mainly due to water retention in the breast tissue accompanied by the breast glands working full-time at starting breastmilk production. If a new mom chooses not to breastfeed or pump, wearing a tight bra and avoiding nipple stimulation can reduce lactation in many.

Breast engorgement can continue till day 7 postpartum. Days 3 to 5 after delivery are usually when the engorgement symptoms peak (the breast fullness, firmness, pain, and tenderness are most intense at this time). The engorgement usually subsides when the breastmilk comes in and your baby is able to have fuller feeds. Or, if you are exclusively pumping, this can help relieve the pain too.

You might experience engorgement from time to time throughout the nursing and pumping period. The engorgement that happens during this time is when the breastmilk supply exceeds the baby's demand or if you're pumping too often.

Abdominal Muscles

The abdominal muscles regain most of their normal muscle tone after several weeks postpartum. Some women regain all of the normal muscle tone. But some experience separation of the rectus muscle, a condition called diastasis recti. Again, postpartum physical rehabilitation is important to check for diastasis recti and to rehabilitate it if present. Without a recovered abdominal wall, there's insufficient core muscle support to improve pelvic floor weakness. See "Pelvic Floor Rehabilitation" in chapter 2 for information on recovery.

Uterus, Cervix, Vagina, and Lochia

The uterus begins to contract as soon as the placenta is delivered to prevent more bleeding. This is called uterine involution. This is why your health providers keep track of where they feel the top of your uterus (the fundus) after you give birth because it usually lies just below the belly button after birth. The uterus should reduce in size every day. It's important for it to keep shrinking to reduce the risk of postpartum haemorrhage. It takes up to 6 to 8 weeks for the uterus to return to pre-pregnancy size (about the size of a pear).

The cervix will remain soft and open after you give birth. After all, it had to dilate up to 10 cm for our baby to exit! Even if you've had a C-section, the cervix will still be dilated to a certain extent and it will definitely remain soft. Just because you had a surgery doesn't mean the cervix skipped the entire labour process. The first few days after giving birth, the cervix usually remains dilated at 2 to 3 cm. By the end of the week, it should be less than 1 cm dilated. However, the cervix opening will not return to its pre-pregnancy shape which is a smooth and circular opening. A cervix that has opened up to deliver a baby will have a long, star-like slit opening once it has recovered.

The vaginal walls are smooth and the vaginal canal is very spacious immediately after delivery. It slowly starts to contract after birth but not as quickly as the uterus. The creases in the vaginal wall are restored around the third week postpartum after excess swelling in the walls have subsided. The vagina does not return completely to its pre-pregnancy size.

Lochia is a substance formed by the shedding of part of the base layer of the placenta after it separates and is delivered. Red or reddish-brown lochia will be discharged in the first few days postpartum. It then usually becomes less red and more yellowish-white. But this is not always the case for every woman. It usually takes 2 to 3 weeks for the lochia to pass but many have passed lochia up to 6 to 8 weeks postpartum. Some even have a bit more to pass after their postpartum check-up. Always ring your health provider if you're unsure whether you're experiencing extended duration of lochia passing. There's no such thing as silly questions when it comes to your bodily functions!

Pelvic Floor

Due to the muscle stretching and overall trauma the pelvic floor endures during childbirth, there's excess pelvic muscle relaxation following delivery, which causes weakness. The pelvic floor muscles do not return to their pre-pregnancy state.

Given the importance of the pelvic floor in supporting the pelvic organs (such as the uterus and bladder), pelvic rehabilitation is crucial in restoring a new mom's pelvic floor health. See "Rehabilitating the Pelvic Floor" in chapter 2 for information on recovery.

Oh my goodness. All that info! Yet, that is actually what YOUR AMAZING BODY is doing while you're also caring for your newborn. Some of you are doing all that while also caring for the rest of the family and trying to go back to work!

CHECK-IN TIME!

How are you feeling now? Amazed? Scared? Horrified? More curious than before?

If you've got more questions from reading the above, write them down! Ask your health providers, your support persons and groups. Go read more if you want! Learn more about your post-birth body however you see fit.

Maybe you also want to take a moment and sit in awe of yourself? Yes, do that. Bookmark this page and put the book down. Do a body scan. Recall your birth experience if you'd like to. Recall your previous postpartum recovery and Postpartum Year experiences. Maybe you're going through it now. And see yourself as I see you, as your children and as your spouse/partner sees you. You're so strong. So indestructible. Yet so very human and full of feelings that are worthy of attention.

You're not alone, dear friend. Not many women and mothers talk about their birth stories or their postpartum journey. And I hope this section of the book helps you see that you can and you should if you want to. You will find others who will listen to your story while

34

> nodding away, happy for the solidarity you bring them.
> And for yourself too!

How insanely formidable is the birthing and post-birth body, right? I'm still in awe of myself till today. I have tremendous respect for every one of you who go through pregnancy, birth, and postpartum once, twice, or many more times.

Yet, these are just the physical changes our body undergoes and "battle scars" we new moms carry for life. There's still the transformation into a mother that's another level of awe which we'll explore in Chapter 2: The Postpartum Journey and Matrescence.

Now, what about the Traditional Chinese Medicine (TCM) approach to postpartum physiology and the Postpartum Year? We'll cover these concepts very briefly to establish a very basic understanding that's sufficient for this book. I recommend that you consult a TCM practitioner for in-depth explanations and tailored consultations. Let's start with some terms you'll come across in this book.

TCM CONCEPTS IN A NUTSHELL

My mother has always cautioned me against Wind and "Cold." And because these concepts have been passed down to her by her mother, just like how she's passed it down to me verbally, we never truly understood why Wind and "Cold" are bad.

All we're told is that they can cause us to feel unwell and predispose us to illness. What kind of illness? According to the advice passed down to my mom and me, well, pretty much everything! Headaches, colds, tummy aches, joint pain and arthritis, low energy, menstrual pain, and bloating, just to name a few.

These ailments are viewed more as signs and symptoms in modern medicine rather than a disease or illness. And once again, I remind you that my grandmother, mother, and myself have been brought up with TCM concepts as laypeople. So, whenever I felt unwell as a kid, I'd just tell my mom I was sick. And that's all we knew.

But now that I've been introduced to TCM knowledge that is written in English (yes, I cannot read or write in Mandarin!), I'm able to satisfy my curiosity about why my mom is so against getting Wind and being "Cold."

Maciocia's textbook *Foundations of Chinese Medicine* is an excellent resource for in-depth reading of TCM principles.[10] For us laypeople who aren't training to become TCM practitioners, a surface overview of the TCM concepts is sufficient for a basic understanding why confinement practices are designed the way they are. So, I've summarised some common TCM concepts according to this textbook.

"Yin" and "Yang"

Over centuries, the concept of "Yin" and "Yang" can be said to be the single most important theory of Chinese medicine. "Yin" and "Yang" hold a similar principle to energy in physics; energy can neither be created nor destroyed, it can only be converted from one form into another. "Yin" and "Yang" are represented by "coolness" and "warmth" respectively. They're always in a state of flux or change. When one increases, the other is "consumed" to preserve balance. This can be observed

---

10. Giovanni Maciocia, *The Foundations of Chinese Medicine: A Comprehensive Text* (Elsevier, 2015).

in the change between night and day, and in the menstrual cycle (bleeding, post-menstrual, ovulation, and pre-menstrual phases). This concept also applies to the body's physiological functions. When the balance is upset, illness abounds. The nature of the illness depends on the degree of excess and depletion of "Yin" (cool) or "Yang" (warm).

Qi

Qi (pronounced "chi") is a core and relatively complex concept in Chinese philosophy and medicine. For an idea of what *Qi* is, I quote Maciocia's text, "Qi is an energy which manifests simultaneously on the physical and emotional-mental-spiritual level."[11] But *Qi* is not the same as "Yin-Yang". To really simplify this difference, think of *Qi* as the internal energy we hold inside us. *Qi* also exists in nature around us and there are many types of *Qi*. Hence, the representations in many Chinese and Chinese-inspired movies where *Qi* can be "absorbed" or "transferred" (kind of like in the *Kung Fu Panda 3* movie where the villain Kai absorbs the *Qi* of many kung fu masters. And their *Qi* is returned to the masters once Kai was defeated). Conversely, "Yin" and "Yang" are the "warmth" and "coolness" that exist within and around us.

Blood

I'll keep this simple. Blood is a form of *Qi*. As Maciocia writes, "Blood is inseparable from *Qi* itself as *Qi* infuses life into Blood; without *Qi*, Blood would be an inert fluid."[12] Blood in Chinese medicine functions to nourish the body. It also forms the foundation for the Mind because it houses

---

11. Maciocia, *The Foundations of Chinese Medicine*, 45.
12. Maciocia, *The Foundations of Chinese Medicine*, 61.

and anchors the Mind. The interesting relation to postpartum mental health is that after blood loss from childbirth any ongoing deficiencies in Blood will cause the Mind to become "unhappy" or "uneasy."

Wind

Wind is "Yang" in nature (warm) and usually "injures" Blood and "Yin". Chinese medicine principles state that Wind carries other harmful climatic factors into the body, such as Cold. Too much Wind in the body can cause convulsions or paralysis. True to how winds behave in nature, many clinical manifestations of Wind start suddenly and can worsen very quickly. It can also cause signs and symptoms of illness to move from one part of the body to another. A common health advice I heard while growing up is that Wind can bring about arthritic pains. In Maciocia's text, there's an explanation that when Wind invades and settles in joints, it can be trapped in there, causing pain, and can also move from one joint to another.[13]

Cold

Cold is "Yin", so it can "injure" "Yang." Why is Cold so bad to have in the body? Cold can congeal Blood, causing Blood stasis. Since Blood is a form of Qi, having stagnant Qi in the body is bad for your overall health. In reproductive health, blood stasis in the uterus is seen as a common cause of painful menses. Cold in the body can also cause stiffness and pain in muscles. If Cold invades the gut, tummy aches and diarrhoea can occur. Cold enters the body via Wind, since Wind is a carrier for many external factors.

---

13. Maciocia, *The Foundations of Chinese Medicine*, 731.

Dampness

Dampness is "Yin" (cooling in nature), so as before, "Yin" tends to "injure" "Yang." Damp living conditions, clothes, skin, and hair are seen as precursors to allowing Dampness to invade the body. Dampness causes things to slow down in the body and is difficult to get rid of. So, during the confinement postpartum recovery month, Dampness is advised to be avoided at all costs to avoid slowing down recovery.[14]

Now that you've got a grasp of these concepts, we'll apply those to the TCM approach to postpartum physiology.

TCM PRINCIPLES REGARDING POSTPARTUM PHYSIOLOGY

In Maciocia's book *Obstetrics and Gynaecology in Chinese Medicine*,[15] he relates the Western term *puerperium* (recall puerperium means the 6–8 weeks the body takes to return to pre-pregnancy state after giving birth) to the Chinese medicine word for the postpartum duration: *chan ru*; *chan* means "childbirth" and *ru* means "cotton mattress."

During this time, there are two main conditions that can occur in the body:

1. **Deficiency of *Qi*, Blood, or "Yin":** During childbirth, we experience blood loss. This negatively affects the Blood and "Yin" elements of the body. Blood loss can lead to blood vessels and channels becoming

---

14. Maciocia, *The Foundations of Chinese Medicine*, 737-8.
15. Giovanni Maciocia, *Obstetrics and Gynecology in Chinese Medicine*, Commissioning Editor: Claire Wilson, Development Editor: Veronika Watkins (Elsevier, 2011), 583-92.

"empty" causing the body to be extremely vulnerable to invasion of Wind. The intensity of delivering a baby also drains a woman's *Qi*.

2. **Blood Stasis:** *Stasis* means "stagnant," or "to stop moving." TCM views that blood stasis after giving birth can occur due to retention of "old blood" in the uterus or retention of lochia.

On top of that, the profuse sweating throughout the labour and birth allows "internal Wind" to develop, and sweating more during the puerperium can damage a woman's *Qi*. The exhaustion of body fluids during birth can also lead to "dryness of the Stomach"[16] causing constipation.

During a call with Dr. Eun Kim, the TCM practitioner who helped me understand the basics of TCM in postpartum health, she explained that the body's "channels" are opened during childbirth as the baby is being born. As imaginable, opened "channels" are very vulnerable to invasion of external factors like Wind, Cold, and Dampness. Since the confinement period is when these "channels" are gradually closing, it's understandable that many confinement practices are aimed at protecting these "channels" from external factors while replenishing internal factors that are depleted. I've been told that our body's "channels" rarely open this wide. So, after giving birth is a good time to make use of widely opened "channels" to rid the body of undesirable factors and boost our internal health!

---

16. Maciocia, *Obstetrics and Gynecology*.

BLAST TO THE PAST: VARIATIONS IN THE POSTPARTUM PERIOD IN CHINESE MEDICINE

Many Chinese medicine texts come from imperial scholars and imperial doctors in the ancient Chinese era. Why? These were mainly the people who had the education and literacy to read, write, and document medical knowledge. Many regular folks would pass knowledge down anecdotally. Additionally, the medical philosophies, practices, and advances in ancient China depended on the ruling dynasty's mission and vision. So, the postpartum period in ancient China varied, including 3 days, 7 days, 1 month, 3 months, 100 days, or up to 1 year after childbirth! This shows that medical terms and knowledge have been evolving and changing since our ancient ancestors' time. So, it makes plenty of sense for us to approach mindsets, medicine, health, science, and technology the same way in our modern world. Otherwise, we can't move forward toward better health goals.

How fascinating was that? I honestly feel like I should've heeded more of my mom's advice when I was younger now that I know what all those TCM terms mean. At least she'll be glad that I'm going to be better at following her Chinese health advice from here on!

Again, you don't need to memorise any of the information in this chapter. You can refer back here anytime as you read the book and prepare for your postpartum recovery.

Chapter 2

The Postpartum Journey and Matrescence

Why is it important to talk about what the postpartum journey is when this book is focused on the postpartum recovery in the early weeks after giving birth?

Because a strong foundation is critical in every adventure and journey we undertake. A solid ship has to be built before setting out on a voyage into the unknown. The postpartum journey is that ship and foundation of many women's motherhood adventures.

Remember that the Postpartum Year includes recovery time in the beginning and the rest of the time needed for our physical, physiological, mental, and emotional sides to adjust to motherhood.

And there's a term for this adjustment period.

WHAT IS MATRESCENCE?

Matrescence: the process of becoming a mother. Matrescence describes the incredible life-altering transition a woman goes through as she becomes a mother. This applies to first-time moms and moms who have more children. This is a developmental phase when physical, psychological, and emotional changes take place, giving rise to identity and relationship changes. Grieving your pre-motherhood self is also recognised as part of matrescence.[17] This grief is described more in chapter 8.

Then why does most of society think that becoming a mother isn't difficult? Why do we, the collective human race, seem to expect mothers to never complain, never ask for help, and just know how to nurse, nurture, and care for new life by ourselves?

Think about it. It's difficult enough for children to become teenagers, for teens to become adults. It's even difficult for some adults to behave like adults.

So, let's move away from the "Supermom" narrative. We don't have to carry the majority of the parenting load. We don't have to know where all the things are. We don't have to remember making all the appointments and buying gifts for special occasions. We don't have to know it all and do it all! Most important, we don't have to be in a constant state of gratitude because, "You chose to have kids!"

While it's flattering and appreciated to have our resiliency recognised, let's also recognise and normalise asking for help and needing help. Let's celebrate being both! To me this is what matrescence is about. A journey into and through motherhood where we'll have wins, losses, and plenty of mountains to climb. And we do it as humans.

---

17. "Why It's Okay to Grieve the Woman You Were Before Motherhood," Shape, last modified October 29, 2020, https://www.shape.com/lifestyle/mind-and-body /grieve-identity-before-motherhood.

A TED talk about matrescence by reproductive psychiatrist Dr. Alexandra Sacks explains this natural process beautifully.[18] I cried the first time I watched it because it answered my deepest question. Oh man, this is normal! This horrid feeling of loss, grief, and disconnect from my identity is NORMAL! The validation I received from the video helped me forgive myself and empowered me to just be human.

BLAST TO THE PAST: THE HISTORY OF MATRESCENCE

Matrescence was first coined by Dana Louise Raphael (1926-2016), an American anthropologist and breastfeeding advocate in the twentieth century. She co-founded the Human Lactation Center where breastfeeding habits of mothers around the world were studied. She was also the first person to use the word *doula* to describe a birthing companion for women in labour.[19]

However, the Chinese cultural views and TCM principles around strong emotions can paint matrescence as a negative thing. I remember growing up with this anecdotal teaching, "Any strong emotion should be avoided at all costs during the confinement period!" I explore more about challenging TCM principles and Chinese cultural traditions around emotions in chapter 8.

---

18. "A new way to think about the transition to motherhood," YouTube video, 6:16, from TED Talk New York in New York on May 2018, posted by "TED", 21 September, 2018, https://www.youtube.com/watch?v=jOsX_HnJtHU.
19. *Doula*: an ancient Greek word meaning "a woman who serves"

THE POSTPARTUM JOURNEY

Since matrescence is a process and a journey, I view it in 4 parts like when I'm taking a flight from one place to another. Each part of the flight will feel different depending on how smooth or rough the journey is.

1. **The Pre-Flight:** Postpartum Planning and Preparation
2. **The Take-Off:** The Modern Confinement Practice and the Fourth Trimester
3. **The Cruising:** The Rest of the Postpartum Year (up to 1 year after childbirth)
4. **The Transit:** Beyond Postpartum Into Motherhood

What can you expect in each part of the journey and how does a modern confinement practice fit in?

The Pre-Flight: Postpartum Planning and Preparation

This usually takes place during the third trimester of pregnancy. There are preparations to make space for the baby at home, baby showers, satisfying the nesting urges, and all other baby-related shopping. But do we give equal attention to preparing the new mom for their recovery weeks? Do we share equal excitement for the first-time mom for their first step into motherhood? Do we actively remember that a mom always cycles back to the "new mom" role with every new addition to the family?

Not often enough!

Our society doesn't do that enough, particularly our modern communities. Our society doesn't truly recognise that new moms need to grow into their new and/or expanding role. Matrescence isn't held with a high value in our modern society's eyes. And this dismissive view flows into the mindset of our employers and local communities, into our family units, and finally into our spouses, partners, family members, and friends.

The modern confinement approach works to reclaim this space and shine the spotlight on the new mom. By taking the time to plan for your postpartum needs and wants, conversations are redirected to you. Your support network is guided to ask questions about what *you* need, not just the baby.

And when new moms prepare their homes, their space, and shop for items to supplement their recovery period, this encourages them to think about how to make things functional for them. Spouses and partners who are directly involved in the planning and preparation can really take a walk in the new mom's shoes. And it encourages them to be selfless for the sake of their loved ones.

The planning stage also encourages new moms to consider boundaries and manage expectations. This is a good time to discuss and set boundaries around visitors during the confinement month and Fourth Trimester, about work and housework, and parenting burden. It's also a good time to manage everyone's expectations about what the confinement month and Fourth Trimester will look and feel like for new moms and their spouses and partners. Chapter 3 takes a deeper dive into this.

Once the pre-flight is complete, it's time for the take-off!

The Take-Off: The Modern Confinement Practice and the Fourth Trimester

You'd think the take-off is about labour and birth. Well, that's just the beginning of the take-off! The engine's got to work extra hard to speed up on the runway and then lift the entire plane up in the air. This. This is labour and birth. You get the buckling down as you work through the contractions during passive labour. Then that huge push just as the plane takes off is akin to active labour. It takes a while to get up off the ground and pull those tires in.

But once the tires are in, the take-off isn't complete yet! There's still the ongoing ascent to reach the cruising altitude. You still gotta keep your seatbelt on, yes? This is where the modern confinement practice comes into play during the Fourth Trimester. This is when new moms will benefit from being nurtured and lifted as they rise into the cruising altitude that is the rest of the Postpartum Year.

WHAT IS THE FOURTH TRIMESTER?

Taking its name from the pregnancy trimesters (more below on Why is it called the Fourth Trimester), the Fourth Trimester is the time between birth and 12 weeks postpartum. Recall that the body's physiological functions (the hormones, muscles, and most other organs and systems in the body) return to pre-pregnancy state about 6 to 8 weeks after giving birth. This is what happens in the Fourth Trimester.[20]

WHY IS IT CALLED THE FOURTH TRIMESTER?

Dr. Harvey Karp, a USA paediatrician and author of *The Happiest Baby* and *Happiest Toddler on the Block* books, coined this term to describe the newborn's transition period from womb to world. He put forth the theory that babies are born too soon at 9 months and so we should "think of babies as fetuses outside

20. "The fourth trimester: What you should know," Harvard Health Publishing, last modified 6 April 2021, https://www.health.harvard.edu/blog/the-fourth-trimester -what-you-should-know-2019071617314.

the womb."[21] Therefore, there's a lot of fussiness and crying to be expected from the baby during these 3 months. The baby really needs their parents to help them adjust to being outside of the warm, snuggly, and dark womb environment.

Once again, although the origin of the Fourth Trimester was developed for newborns, there's growing support on using the same term and duration to focus on supporting a new mom's postpartum health. Why not? After all, we've got to nurture the nurturer first before they can provide for the baby! Place the oxygen mask on yourself before aiding others with theirs, correct?

The modern confinement practice ties into the Fourth Trimester as the first 4 weeks of nurturing the new mom out of the Fourth Trimester's 12 weeks. Boosting the recovery in the first month after giving birth ensures that new moms have the energy to recover and have enough energy reserve for daily functions such as caring for the household and family, nursing and feeding the baby, and going back to work early for some. This modern confinement month can also give space to new moms to build a foundation on which to continue their recovery journey for the remainder of the Fourth Trimester.

This is the time to settle in your new mom's pilot seat and let the computer systems do their thing with the take-off. And lean on your co-pilot(s)! Your spouse, partner, family members, and friends. You just need to set the travel path and let your support systems and network help you keep your hands on the flight controls.

---

21. "What Is the Fourth Trimester?" Happiest Baby Blog, last modified date unavailable, https://www.happiestbaby.com/blogs/baby/fourth-trimester.

Once the modern confinement practice is completed and the Fourth Trimester has passed, what can new moms expect for the rest of the Postpartum Year?

The Cruising Altitude: 3–12 Months Postpartum

Now that the seat belt lights are off, you can get up and move about the aeroplane! Turbulence will occur every now and then, but you'll get used to it. The rest of the Postpartum Year will have you enjoying the flight and then suddenly being forced to endure some rough turbulence whether you're sitting down in your seat or standing up doing something.

There's the baby's fussiness during growth spurts and teething, and even a toddler's tantrums due to having to adjust to a new family member. We're worried for them—yet also annoyed, exhausted, and frustrated at being terribly sleep deprived. We're overstimulated by all the noise and neediness. Yet we feel fulfilled because only we can give our children the comfort they need. Our children come to us to feel safe.

Then there are the emotional changes you'll go through as the postpartum hormones settle into a new or pre-pregnancy pattern. And these changes don't stop with the hormones. Because one random day, we might yearn for the days before we had children. *"Gosh, what was it even like? Why can't I really remember?"* And of course, guilt will come and shame us for thinking such things. For wanting to go back to being the person we were before we had all this responsibility of keeping a small human alive.

Because of that, some of us feel sick and tired of having our days revolve around the baby, barely having any down time for ourselves. There are those of us who can't wait to put some distance between us, baby, and being at home all the time. So touched out, so overwhelmed.

Some of us must go back to work and that's a horribly rough time to part with our baby before we're ready. We miss the ability to just play and snuggle with our babies whenever we want and not worry about having to be well-rested for a workday tomorrow. Some of us still want to enjoy nursing our baby, watching them watch us as they smile and coo at the breast. And somehow, during this tender moment, a sob and tear escapes you. *"Oh, how innocent and carefree you are right now! Yet our world will be cruel to you as you grow up."*

And as suddenly as those heavy thoughts come, they're replaced by a sense of awe and wonder at what we've achieved. We've just brought new life into this world! Our babies are not only alive, they're thriving! Thriving! *"Oh, I must be doing something right!"* Yes, yes we are! Despite all our flaws and still having to deal with our inner child traumas.

Why Preparation Matters

So, how does applying a modern confinement practice at the start of matrescence help in this stage? Having a whole month to focus on yourself also allows you to spend time snuggling your newborn. With help from your support network, be it familial or hired, there's so much relief from the mental and physical load. You're able to be more present and can actually enjoy your time in recovery!

With this rejuvenation, the rest of the Postpartum Year becomes more manageable. You'll still hit the ground running but you'll have your fuel tanks replenished. The physical and emotional tanks. And on bad days, you'll be more open to asking for help and receiving it. Because you've done it before! And you know you're not alone in your postpartum journey.

If your partner, spouse, and older children were involved in your modern confinement month, they'd know that when you need help, you NEED help. They're likely to have more appreciation and empathy for you having cared for you through your most vulnerable period. And they know they'll do a good job of helping you too! All of you would've built trust for each other during the modern confinement month. This can go a long way in the rest of your postpartum journey and set a wonderful example for your children (boys and girls alike) that raising a family is best done as a team.

The Transit: Beyond Postpartum into Motherhood

Is there an end to matrescence? I propose the answer, "No!"

Why? Recall the description of matrescence at the beginning of this chapter, "This is a developmental phase when physical, psychological, and emotional changes take place, giving rise to identity and relationship changes."

As a mom transitions along with their baby from newborn to infant, and then toddlerhood, childhood, adolescence, and beyond, there's a shift in the parent identity, including psychological and emotional changes with each stage! This constant state of flux in a mom's identity needs to be recognised as an integral part of their life course so that we can provide appropriate support at the appropriate time.

Therefore, I view things as "in transit" after the Postpartum Year. We're just in a transit lounge waiting to board the next flight to Toddlerland or Teenagewoods. We don't cease being parents once our kids become adults either. They're still our children regardless of how old they are! Then some of us might hop on to Grandparentworld!

Now that we've mapped out the postpartum journey, let's discuss other useful things about postpartum care.

WHAT'S IMPORTANT IN POSTPARTUM CARE?

Postpartum care varies across the globe. Since I expect you, dear reader, to hail from anywhere in the world, I won't be delving into what's offered in each country. What I'll encourage you to do is to find out what kind of postpartum services you're entitled to and how to access them.

You've got to take the proactive approach here. Ask your health providers and insurance companies. I understand health insurance plays a big part in many countries, so get to know what yours offers, if you have one. Talk to government health centres and nonprofit organisations in your area. Always ask when in doubt! If someone doesn't know the answer, ask who else you could talk to. You'd be amazed how much information you get just by asking around and how much help can be available to you. Then, you can plan your needs around what's available to you!

Here are some key postpartum topics to think about and discuss with your loved ones and/or health providers.

Delaying Baby's First Bath after Birth

When clinical staff talk about delaying your newborn's first bath, it's due to recent updates in understanding the role of the vernix. The vernix is made up of water, fats, and proteins to form a protective white film over your baby's skin while still in the womb. After all, our baby is fully immersed and suspended in amniotic fluid for months! This protective barrier prevents your baby's skin from breaking down while inside the uterus.

This practice should already be followed by your health providers. But for your peace of mind, do remind them if you'd like to delay your baby's first bath. How long? The recommendation is for 6 to 24 hours after birth. For me, I really loved the way my firstborn smelled, like a light hint of fresh flowers and well, the baby smell! I wanted to keep sniffing her baby-ness forever. Of course, they wiped her down so that she wouldn't get chilly in the air-conditioned birth suite. But they didn't clean off the vernix completely.

I only allowed them to bathe her the next day because I didn't want her to lose that baby smell. I didn't have a similar experience with my second baby because I had an emergency C-section and I honestly don't remember much!

Now, the good thing about leaving the vernix on your baby for those hours is the ongoing temperature regulation it provides to your baby's tiny body. It helps maintain their core temperature by allowing their small body to gradually adjust to their new environmental temperature. Remember, your young one was literally thrust out into our cold and dry world (if you're in an air-conditioned birth suite or in a dry climate country). All they knew before that was a warm, buoyant, and comfortable bubble!

There's also an evolving theory that leaving the vernix on your baby's skin helps with breastfeeding and nursing success for those who want to nurse. The idea is that bathing your baby later will allow more skin-to-skin time with mom, increasing the bond between both. And yes, skin-to-skin time is highly recommended between baby and fathers/partners too! The vernix also supposedly smells just like the amniotic fluid, the only scent your baby ever knew up till being born. So, having this familiar scent linger for hours after birth while doing skin-to-skin time is thought to encourage your baby to latch better onto the nipple should you choose to breastfeed. And since everything smells so comforting, your baby might be more successful at latching—or at least they won't mind trying hard!

Rehabilitating the Pelvic Floor

This is very important. Why? Our women's health is inextricably tied to our uterus and ovaries, our menstrual cycle, and our hormones. Rehabilitation for our reproductive organ and its supporting structures after birth is important for our physical, mental, and sexual health.

WHAT IS THE PELVIC FLOOR?

The pelvic floor is made up of muscles that stretch from the pubic bone to the tailbone. This "floor" of muscles supports the bladder, lower intestines, vagina, and uterus in women. When the muscle floor is working properly, all those organs stay in place and help them function properly. The pelvic floor muscles also support the growing womb but it has to relax as the pregnancy progresses to prepare for labour and birth. The pelvic floor's strength is further supported by our core muscles, including the abdominal muscles.

Why does the pelvic floor need rehabilitation after birth? All pregnant women will experience a weakened pelvic floor after birth. This is due to the hormonal changes that directly instruct the muscles to relax so that birth can occur as smoothly as possible. The rectus abdominis (the abdominal core muscle that we usually refer to as "abs") can separate during pregnancy. And for some of us, this separation persists a few months after we've given birth, causing diastasis recti. We need all these muscles to return to their pre-pregnancy function as best as possible so that we don't end up with life-long issues such as the following:

- Urinary leakage or unable to control bladder
- Painful sex
- Constipation or unable to control bowel movements
- Lower back pain
- Pelvic pains, including pain in the rectum and vagina

When untreated, these problems worsen in old age risking a condition called "pelvic organ prolapse." This is when the pelvic organs (uterus, intestines, and bladder) "drop down" from their normal position and bulge into the vagina passageway. This visual is enough to make anyone squirm in discomfort!

Yet, many women are told it's "normal" to experience all the above issues after giving birth. Sure, it's COMMON, but it shouldn't be dismissed as normal! So, mothers should NEVER be told, "That's just how it is," or "You just have to put up with it," when there are programs available.

It's been difficult for me, honestly, to have urinary leakage at only 30 years old, and constantly worrying if I'll smell like pee when I'm around others. Wearing pads and panty liners all the time has been rough on my vulvar skin too. So, after both my kids, I asked my OBGYN to refer me for pelvic rehab therapy since my insurance didn't automatically include pelvic rehab after giving birth (I had a USA health insurance when I had both my kids). Thankfully, my insurance covered them once my OBGYN put in a referral. But if you're in Germany or France and have access to their healthcare services, then you're in luck! Pelvic rehab for all women after giving birth is considered standard postpartum care there.

What does pelvic floor rehab involve?

Pelvic floor rehabilitation aims to restore function to the weakened pelvic floor muscles and the other muscle groups that support it. In turn, this helps the pelvic organs remain where they are in the pelvis and reduce those postpartum issues mentioned above.

But this isn't just about doing Kegel exercises. This also isn't about following trainers and gurus on social media. While some do have good tips, it's still important to see a physical therapist to identify exactly what your pelvic floor needs. More importantly, a physical therapist specialising in pelvic floor injuries should be assessing you after you've recovered from the birth. This is their domain of expertise after all. Ideally, this is done after your 6- or 8-week postpartum checkup or after you've recovered from any injuries or surgery.

Firstly, the physical therapist will usually teach you how to identify where your pelvic muscles are and how they feel when you're contracting and relaxing them. The easiest way to do this accurately is through the vagina, either manually with fingers or with a small probe that measures muscle contraction and relaxation. This is crucial so that you know that you're exercising the right muscles at home. However, if you're uncomfortable with being examined this way, please let your physical therapist know. They can then recommend other ways to teach you how to feel the pelvic floor muscles in action.

Then you'll learn exercises to strengthen and stabilise the abdominal core muscles, back muscles, pelvic floor, and the diaphragm. Yes! The diaphragm is also very important in pelvic floor rehab.

WHAT IS THE DIAPHRAGM?

This is a thin muscle that sits at the bottom of your chest. It separates the chest from the abdomen. It flattens when you take a deep breath in (Let's do it now. Breathe in deeply and feel your belly rise) because your lungs are expanding and pushing this muscle layer down. So, following the domino effect, that means your abdominal organs and pelvic floor are also pushed down. When you exhale, the diaphragm contracts and so everything below it comes back up.

The rehab is slow and results are also slow to show. But that's to be expected! Your body literally rearranged its insides and your joints expanded over the course of about 9 months. It will take time for your muscles to mosey their way back. And you should be taking it slow, otherwise those muscles are going to get more stressed and recover slower instead.

So, I highly encourage you to speak to your health practitioner about postpartum pelvic floor rehabilitation, especially if you're living in a country that does not offer this as a standard of postpartum care.

Be straightforward when asking for it. Be up front with the issues you're having. Tell them sex is painful if that's exactly what's happening. Tell them you're having urinary leakage when you laugh, cough, or sneeze. Tell them about your lower back pains. You deserve to know if these problems are due to pelvic floor injuries from the birth and to get that seen proactively instead of waiting it out. And remember, if you're questioned (if you hear "Why do you want a referral, it's normal?"), NO, IT'S NOT!

> *Tip:* If you feel like your concerns are not taken seriously, seek out the clinic or hospital's patient liaison person. Or someone with the capacity to advocate for you in a healthcare setting. This position and person varies across countries. Start by asking the clinic receptionist, a ward's nurse unit manager, or a social worker if you're not sure where to start!

Forging a Good Relationship with Your Health Providers

Throughout this book, I'll always advise you to see a TCM practitioner to discuss your unique situation and needs, especially if you're seeking herbal concoctions to consume during the confinement month. While there are generic recipes out there sold by herbal and confinement companies, it's always best to get a TCM prescription specific to you.

But there's a limitation for what TCM can do for you. In the case of fevers, bleeding, bloody lochia that doesn't seem to be resolving, and pain that feels out of proportion to you for having already given birth, it's important to seek your modern health provider immediately. Even TCM practitioners today will advise their patients to see modern medical doctors to ensure no life-threatening conditions are brewing before prescribing TCM treatments.

In my modernising of the confinement practice, I view TCM practitioners as supporting the new mom during their recovery period once they're cleared of any danger from the modern medical health provider. TCM practitioners are experts in herbal concoctions and complementary therapies like acupuncture for pain management and *gua sha* massage for lymphatic drainage. They'll know how much of these treatments you'll need during your confinement month and after. They can also help with lactation issues like regulating milk supply and mastitis management. Very similar to Western-trained lactation educators and consultants. However, if you ever start feeling very, very sick (symptoms can vary from fainting, nausea, sweats, chills, racing heart, and terrible pain), see your modern medical health provider immediately!

At the same time, I also recommend discussing your herbal consumption with your modern health practitioners because if you've got certain health conditions or are on certain medications, it's wise to find out whether the herbal concoctions are safe to consume while on treatment. So if there's any conflicting medications or conditions, your TCM practitioner can alter your herbal prescriptions and advise you accordingly.

Trusting that you can discuss anything with your health practitioners is very important for your mental health after giving birth. As a pregnant woman, first-time mom, or a new mom of an expanding family in many modern societies, sometimes our main support is our health practitioner. Not all of us live close to family and friends these days, so we're not always able to lean on them. The risk and ease of spread of global pandemics has further dampened the ability for loved ones to come together to help new moms. I encourage you to allow yourself to form a good relationship with your health practitioners so that you can go to them anytime. If your health insurance or finances allow, find a therapist or counsellor too. They're a good point of contact to vent to when your family and friends aren't able to help.

DECIDING IF YOUR HEALTH PROVIDER IS RIGHT FOR YOU

Yes, you do have the right to change providers if you're not jiving with them. Why? It's important to feel comfortable to ask any questions and bring up any concerns without worrying about being judged or dismissed. This is good for your health! Here are a few things to consider:

- *Language:* Naturally, without speaking the same language, it's going to be difficult to develop a close relationship! Mistranslations, misunderstandings, and miscommunications risk happening more than usual. I recommend finding a provider who speaks your first language. This is also important so that you don't have to bring a family member or friend as a translator if you want to discuss something private.
- *How do they hold space for complementary therapies?* If you'd like to try complementary therapies, how do they respond when you discuss it with them? Do they scoff at Reiki and dismiss your interest in trying it? Or do they support you in wanting to give alternative or complementary therapies a go to supplement your recovery? Especially if they themselves don't fully agree with the treatment principles. From my professional past as a medical doctor, I found that holding space for my patients and their families to explore complementary therapies brought us closer as a team. And it helped

them feel a lot more comfortable approaching me to discuss anything they'd like because I had put their beliefs and needs first.

- *A good listener:* Hearing and listening are two different things. Yes, they are. The words themselves describe two different events. Listening is intentional. Hearing is not. Listening is an action. Hearing is not. When we say, "Do you hear me?" we usually mean, "Can you hear me speak clearly?" When we say, "Are you listening to me?" we usually mean, "Are you giving me undivided attention to fully understand why I'm worried?" You know you have a provider who listens well when you leave their office feeling good. Light. Understood. Even if they hadn't cured or solved your problem entirely!
- *Someone who validates your concerns:* No matter how big, small, or serious your worries seem to your provider, a good one will validate them for you. They will confirm that your worries are legitimate, no matter what. You'll feel safe to fret in their presence, instead of feeling like you're just being dramatic. They'll remind you that you're not crazy. If your anxiety and concerns are truly out of proportion, they will still validate your feelings and then guide you toward the help you need. They'll see you when you need to be seen more than ever before.

Consulting with a TCM Practitioner

Many TCM practitioners nowadays are very good at working with modern medicine. I highly recommend consulting with one while you're pregnant so that you can plan for your confinement month in advance. This allows you to discuss and prepare for any complications or worries that you and your modern health practitioner might have about the Postpartum

Year. It's also worth asking for an herbal concoction that is safe to consume after a C-section, since there's always a chance for an emergency C-section to occur!

I once visited a TCM practitioner who specialises in women's health in Malaysia prior to having my first kid. I wanted her to assess my overall health and help me prepare for trying for a baby. (No, I wasn't having fertility issues, but I have a history of irregular menses and wanted some TCM input about my female health since I grew up with TCM.) Once we confirmed from my medical history that I didn't have any women's health conditions that required modern medicine intervention, she requested a pelvis ultrasound to assess the structure of my ovaries and uterus. Only after this did she complete her assessment and prescribe me some herbs to take after each menses (the common generic recipe is called *pak cheng*). My mother used to brew this for me to drink after my menses was complete and, boy, did I dislike drinking it as a teenager!

When I was pregnant with my first child and living in the USA, I also consulted a TCM practitioner there so that I could get the correct herbs for my confinement needs. He took a thorough medical history from me including the input from my OBGYN. The herbal department pharmacist also taught my husband how to brew the herbs.

Even though I'm a medical doctor trained in modern medicine, I'm still a Malaysian who grew up using both modern medicine and TCM. So, I really loved my TCM experiences of rejuvenating my body after menses and preparing for my confinement month. The TCM practitioners I've met have showed me how relevant TCM has become to our twenty-first century world.

Feeding Your Baby

Why There's Minimal Breastfeeding and Nursing Advice in This Book

I don't discuss breastfeeding much in this book because I personally find that nursing is an art and not every person enjoys it. I didn't at first because I had horrible mini panic attacks every time before my milk let down. Imagine feeling an impending sense of doom every time baby nurses; every day, every session, day and night. I had that for a whole year even while on antidepressants for my postpartum depression and anxiety (the meds just dulled the panic feeling; they didn't remove it completely).

My lactation consultant told me I had D-MER (Dysphoric Milk Ejection Reflex) where instead of the fluffy happy feeling that usually accompanies breastfeeding, I was experiencing negative emotions.

What Is D-MER?

D-MER is a term coined by Alia Macrina Heise and Diane Wiessinger (both are IBCLCs—International Board-Certified Lactation Consultants) that describes a physiological reaction toward breastfeeding, specifically during let-downs (the milk ejection reflex). Unlike the "euphoria" felt by many who nurse, those with D-MER experience the opposite.

D-MER can bring about feelings of anxiety, depression, sadness, irritability, and restlessness right before the let-down occurs. It can take between 30 seconds to 2 minutes for feelings to subside.

Currently, there isn't a "cure" for this phenomenon except time. Most who nurse find that the intense feelings gradually lessen over time as they continue nursing. They may linger for the entire breastfeeding period. For some, their D-MER eventually goes away completely.

History of D-MER

Heise and Wiessinger first published their findings in 2011 in the *International Breastfeeding Journal*.[22] Before this, there were very few resources (almost none!) on what this horrible feeling was and how to manage it. Heise started a blog and website dedicated to her experience with D-MER to document her journey, connect and support others with D-MER, and collect more information on the phenomenon.

Since publishing their paper on D-MER, Heise and Wiessinger hope that scientific researchers working with hormones such as dopamine will study this phenomenon in more depth.

D-MER Resources

I highlight this condition in my book so that if you think you have D-MER during your confinement month (or if you as a support person notice this about your loved ones), know that you're not imagining things. You're not a bad mother. You're not being dramatic. This is a real condition. Your hormones are controlling many aspects of your Postpartum Year, including your behaviour!

Heise has also written a book about this condition and phenomenon. So, instead of me covering D-MER in detail, I encourage you to read her book and visit the website for in-depth explanations and recommendations on managing D-MER.

22. Alia M. Heise, Diane Wiessinger, "Dysphoric milk ejection reflex: A case report," *International Breastfeeding Journal* volume 6, Article Number 6 (2011), https://doi.org/10.1186/1746-4358-6-6.

- **Website:** www.D-MER.org
- **Facebook group:** Dysphoric Milk Ejection Reflex (D-MER) Support Group from d-mer.org
- **Heise's self-published book:** *Before The Letdown—Dysphoric Milk Ejection Reflex and the Breastfeeding Mother* (2017)

I had to really differentiate D-MER from my postpartum depression and anxiety symptoms every time I nursed my baby. It took a lot of mental and emotional fortitude to deal with that on a daily basis. But at least I knew what was happening and that helped me take better control of the situation.

It's important to connect with your local breastfeeding consultants, lactation educators, fellow nursing mothers, and nursing support groups. Those of us with breasts (or to be anatomically correct: functional lactating glands on our chests) are still expected to "naturally" know how to breastfeed and nurse. Unfortunately, that's not the case and we need all the help we can get!

The Pressures and Conflicts of Breastfeeding

While it's great to breastfeed and nurse our babies, not everyone with breasts and lactating glands can do it. Sometimes, the glands are just unable to produce enough milk. So, supplementing with formula is the best thing for your baby. But what about way back in the olden days when formula wasn't invented yet? What else was there besides animal milk, flour, and sugar?

Wet nurses! Wet nurses are lactating women and persons who are able to produce good amounts of breastmilk to feed their babies and others' babies. It was common for wealthier families to have wet nurses feed their babies, especially someone to look after babies overnight. Naturally, there's a whole history behind wet nurses: socio-economic classes, racism, and slavery. To discuss these aspects is out of the scope of this book. I encourage you to look it up at your own time if you're interested in learning more.

But my mother, aunties, and many others in their generation largely entered motherhood with the notion that breastfeeding and nursing should come "naturally" to all women. My mom and aunts told me that they didn't really have anyone to teach them about baby latching basics, how to manage breast and gland engorgement, and how to manually express milk. The pressure was there to "just know how to do it."

My mom and aunts said the initial nursing days were too painful for them to bear and they didn't have enough milk. So, they fed my generation formula. Thank goodness for that! I can't begin to imagine the guilt and despair the ladies in my family would've felt if they couldn't feed us. Yet, as time went by, those of us who chose formula-feeding (or had to use formula) over breastfeeding were still judged.

But what if we choose to not breastfeed at all? Is that bad? Good? Responsible? Irresponsible?

Frankly, it really isn't anyone's business whether we feed our babies with formula, breastmilk, or both. Or why we make that decision.

The main question to ask yourself if you're ever feeling unsure is, "Is my baby growing well and healthy on formula, breastmilk, and/or both?"

When you answer, "YES!" that means you're doing a wonderful job!

Will this pressure and judgement ever end?

Sadly, I don't think it will for generations. The best we can do now is to be confident in our choices on how we want to feed our babies. We can choose to be the cycle breaker for our children's generation. This includes setting boundaries on how much judgement we will tolerate and how we want to respond.

Breastfeeding Resources

- **La Leche League International:** I recommend searching online or asking around your local community about local La Leche League groups. There are many globally!

- **IBCLCs in your local area:** IBCLCs are International Board Certified Lactation Consultants that work independently or with organisations and agencies. The process to becoming an IBCLC can be gruelling due to the requirement that all IBCLCs must have a Health Sciences education and longer contact hours before certification is granted. Now you know how to search for these qualified lactation experts in your area!

- **Lactation Consultants or Educators:** Similar to IBCLCs, these professionals provide lactation education and support to breastfeeding moms. The certification process is different from IBCLCs and varies depending on the organisation that provides the training. Again, you can search online or within your community for these consultants in your local area.

Why There Isn't Formula Feeding Advice in This Book

I won't be making any recommendations on formula brands or types. I won't be discussing the ins and outs of formula feeding either. Why? This book is focused on the new mom. Not on the newborn. Instead, I'll make recommendations on how a new mom can organise their home and postpartum plan to make formula feeding easier to manage. For advice on formula feeding, please refer to your baby's health professional(s).

MANAGING EXPECTATIONS IN THE POSTPARTUM YEAR

This part of postpartum care deserves an entire chapter dedicated to it. Managing expectations comes with setting boundaries. This combination can play a huge role in improving and maintaining a new mom's mental and emotional health. So hop on to the next chapter for a deep dive! Key things to remember:

- Always check what postpartum care you're entitled to in your country and under your insurance. Talk to your health practitioners about what you need and how to access it.
- Get in on some postpartum pelvic rehabilitation! This applies to after vaginal and C-section births.
- Always consult both your modern and TCM health practitioners with any doubts. Provide both of them with each other's contact details. Whether they consult with each other is up to them. Doing your best to keep the conversation going between everyone ensures your and your baby's safety and health in the Postpartum Year!

Chapter 3

Managing Expectations and Setting Boundaries in the Postpartum Year

"How can you say you don't want to follow these traditions? It's for your own good!"

"If you don't follow these rules properly, you'll get all sorts of problems later and when you're old."

"Don't ask so many questions. This is how it's always been done."

"Stop complaining. I didn't complain when I had to follow all these rules."

"I don't really trust what the modern doctor says. I think follow the Chinese sensei better."

Talk about unsolicited advice! And unfortunately, some of our moms and mothers-in-law (MILs) will give their opinions regardless of how that makes you feel. They can do it directly in your face or passive aggressively. The "tsk tsk!" or loud sighs when you're not doing something the way they like it. Or they may make passing comments just loud enough for you to hear.

"Bao Bei, *why are you always hungry? Your mother didn't feed you enough, is it?"* they might say to the baby despite you already explaining that bubba is having a growth spurt.

Ugh. Just. UGH.

That said, there must be a way for us to retain some sanity during this vulnerable time. If our body needs physical nourishment to recover, our minds and hearts should also receive the same tender nourishment.

It's easier said than done to heed the sentiment, "Oh, just let them be. They're old."

Or, "Oh, just let it 'one ear in, one ear out'. Ignore them!"

So, dear new moms, let's take a dive into how to manage our expectations of ourselves and others around us during the Postpartum Year. This will start allowing us to set boundaries comfortably and confidently. And most important, be GUILT-FREE about it!

ELDERS AND TRADITION

Why Do Our Elders Take the Confinement Practice So Seriously?

First, let's visit a few concepts that give us a glimpse into why our elders can be so strict about keeping to confinement traditions and why they might behave in a certain way with new parents, especially moms.

Culture and Tradition

Naturally, our moms and/or MILs would have been expected to follow the confinement tradition and certain cultural practices unique to their spouse's family when they were new moms back in their days. A very traditional motivator for observing the confinement month is to care for the new mother so that they can bear more kids. It was all about continuing the paternal lineage. This belief still exists in many families and cultures in the twenty-first century.

But there's no doubt that our elders faced very similar uncertainties, insecurities, and worries as we do as new moms today. They might also have wanted to do things their way but didn't have the confidence and support to speak up. So, the trickle-down effect we get can sound like, "It's always been done this way," or "Don't ask so many questions; just follow the rules."

Generational Difference

There's also a generational difference when it comes to trust in healthcare providers. Many Asian elders I knew grew up with Traditional Chinese Medicine and other local health treatments in their town or village. Herbs and concoctions were the go-to for many ailments. Acupuncture, cupping, and massages were commonly prescribed treatments. It's also important to understand that many Asian countries didn't have a great outcome under British and Western colonisers. Naturally, many medical advancements and modern lifestyle changes that were deemed "Western" were not easily embraced and trusted.

I've definitely heard many older Malaysians (regardless of ethnicity) say, "I don't want to see Western doctors. They always find problems and give me pills that make me feel worse." My grandfather said that. He passed away in 2005 after a few years of suffering from 2 strokes and a heart bypass surgery. This sentiment still holds firm today. My mom, aunts, and uncles in Malaysia would rather follow Traditional Chinese Medicine principles than modern medicine. The irony? I'm a modern medically trained physician.

So, to our elders, following the confinement practice after giving birth is of utmost importance to ensure the new mom's health is preserved and rejuvenated so that they can provide the best for baby—and to prevent health issues in old age. To go against this can be blasphemy for many elders.

But what does this look like in terms of behaviour from your mom, mother-in-law, or a hired confinement support person who is an elder from the previous generation?

Behaviour You Might Encounter during Confinement from an Elder

Taking Over Your Kitchen

If you're having your mom and/or MIL come stay with you during or after the confinement month, it might feel like they're always in your kitchen doing something. That can be great because that means you and your spouse or partner may not have to do any cooking or cleaning up. But that can also feel like your autonomy is being taken away because it can come across as not having access to your kitchen anymore. It can also feel like because they're the one cooking and stocking up your kitchen, things are rearranged to suit them. You may also feel like you're not able to have any food, drink, or snack you want at any time of the day because it might seem like they're hovering over your shoulder and judging your food and drink choices. But bear in mind that they're probably not consciously doing any judging or trying to take over your home. It can come across that way because you and your spouse or partner are used to being independent and having your home all to yourself until now.

Rearranging Things in Your Home

Just like how they might rearrange things in your kitchen, they might do the same to other parts of your home because they're there to help with all other chores during the confinement month. Chances are, they'll put things where it's convenient for them and where they think it'll be convenient for you. Again, this can be great because you and your spouse or partner may not need to do these chores while you recover and settle into your growing family. Once again, this can start to feel like your elder is taking over your home because having a parent come stay with you as an adult child feels very different from when we stayed with our parents as kids and teenagers.

Barging into Your Room without Knocking

Since they're here to look after you and your newborn, chances are you've automatically given up your privacy during the confinement month. Your mom and/or MIL might just come into your and your spouse or partner's room without knocking when the baby starts crying. Or they might just come in when they want to serve you food and beverages, or to check on you. Again, this can be great! Breakfast, lunch, and dinner in bed! But, man, this lack of privacy can be overwhelming. It already feels like they've taken over your entire home and now, you can't even have this sliver of privacy? Gosh!

Sidelining Your Partner

Remember that our elders grew up during a time where many fathers and males barely got involved in any nurturing roles.

Their husbands and fathers were unlikely to change diapers, soothe a crying baby, feed a baby, or bathe and change a baby. It's unlikely the men in their lives would often step up and offer to give moms a break. So naturally, if your mom and/or MIL comes to stay with you during your confinement month, they might expect your male spouse or partner to "stay out of the way" so that they can focus on you, the newborn, and the home. They'll likely jump in to take a crying baby from your male spouse or partner because they'll assume he doesn't know how to soothe the baby. Or that he'd have the patience to try. This can be very frustrating for male spouses and partners for many reasons. Here are just two:

1. **Male spouses and partners feel like they're looked down upon:** Having your own child taken from you for basic things like soothing, feeding, bathing, and diaper changing can send a message that "you don't know what you're doing," and "you're not a fit parent." For many spouses and partners (regardless of gender and sex), not being able to look after their family can feel very degrading and embarrassing. And powerless. Male spouses and partners already can't do much physically during their loved one's labour and birth, so to take this away from them is akin to stripping them of the final sliver of ability they have to help their family.

2. **Male spouses and partners feel like they're excluded from their own new and growing family:** I suppose this is how many new moms can feel when the baby is here. When all the focus is on the newborn, the new mom is easily reduced to being a human vessel of sustenance and nurturing. Male spouses and partners

can also feel this way because they're traditionally fully excluded from the Postpartum Year and nurturing of children. It's "always been a woman's and female's role." But modern fathers and male spouses and partners are turning the tables on this damaging aspect of patriarchy. They want to be involved! They want to be there for the pregnancy, labour, and birth. They want to be there for their loved ones' postpartum recovery. They want to change the diapers and soothe their crying newborn all night. They want to cook the confinement foods and prepare the confinement teas and soups. So, for elders to behave in ways that don't allow male spouses and partners to take part in the confinement month is akin to excluding them from their own family. As though they don't matter at all during this time.

Doing Things Their Way with Your Baby

Since our elders have "done it all before," it's likely they'll do things their way with regards to caring for your baby. However, there are many changes to infant care since modern medicine and research have shown us different and sometimes, safer, ways of doing things. But recall the discussion at the beginning of this chapter on generational differences and views on traditional versus modern medicine. They might say, "Oh, I did this when so-and-so was a baby and look, they turned out fine!" They could also think of you as giving them rules to follow about infant care, as if they didn't know any better. And with them being elders in a traditional sense, they may not take kindly to that.

Giving Unsolicited Comments and Advice

Oh this. As much as physical behaviours can irk us, these unsolicited words can cut deeper. Our elders can make comments on everything. From how we're changing our baby to how we're sitting on the couch with the baby. From what we eat to how we're eating our food. There will very likely be comments on our postpartum bodies and looks although we've just given birth: "Oh, you're so swollen!" or "Wow, you lost so much weight so quickly!" The latter might sound like praise, but too quick weight loss isn't always a good thing because our bodies have adapted to the pregnancy weight over 9 months. And there's the seed planted in our minds that "Oh, I gotta keep up this tremendous weight loss moving forward! How amazing will it be to have bounced back so quickly!" Even well-meaning comments to our male spouses and partners like, "Oh wow, you can change a diaper!" can come across as condescending. I mean, who wants to be viewed as so "useless" that even learning how to change a diaper is such an amazing feat?

Merging Generational Expectations

We cannot control or expect our moms and mothers-in-law (MILs) to change their behaviours. They've grown up in a completely different era with very restricting social views of women, mothers, and females. This is especially true for our elders in Asian countries. Many of our female elders also don't always share their history, so they might have unresolved trauma and may project those onto us.

A lot of conflicting exchanges between the new mother and their mom or MIL during the confinement period are also emotional rather than logical or rational. So, addressing emotions with data and science usually isn't successful. What we can do is understand where they might be coming from (but that does not excuse bad behaviour!) so that we can adjust our expectations, set boundaries, and manage our reactions. We have the best control over ourselves, so let's work with that strength.

To be closest to success, you'll need to get creative with finding solutions that will appease both your emotions and your elder's emotions. Work with your spouse or partner, friends, and other family members, especially those who know your mom and/or MIL well. That'll increase the chance of your mom and/or MIL accepting your wish for a modern confinement month.

Remember, you and your spouse or partner are human. As empathetic as you try to be, you're bound to want to say a few things if you're experiencing rude behaviours from your elders during your confinement month or while you're planning it.

WHY DO WE TALK ABOUT APPEASING BOTH SIDES IN THIS CHAPTER?

This is the burden of being a cycle breaker. We've got this chance to show our elders that we can be modern yet respectful of tradition and culture. And we're setting an example for the younger generation that we can respect and follow tradition in a modern way. So, yes, I recommend coming up with ideas on how to rope our elders in to come along for this modern confinement practice. We'll talk about these ideas later in this chapter. But if you don't want to do this, that's okay too. It's your call or your and your spouse's/partner's collective decision.

FILIAL PIETY

You might feel many emotions while combating generational expectations, most of all GUILT. You'll feel straight up GUILTY AS HECK in the beginning for not wanting to follow the confinement rules as strictly as your mom and/or MIL says you should. This guilt can come on very strongly for those of us who grew up in Asian households that uphold the concept of filial piety.

The concept of filial piety is an interesting one. Understanding this will help tremendously in coming up with ideas on how to broach the topic of guiding your elders toward compromising on a modern confinement month. The root of filial piety lies in ancestor worship during a time when Chinese emperors believed that they were descendants of Shang Di, "the great founder ancestor god."[23] Thus, worshipping ancestors and making sacrifices in their honour would bless the current emperor with guidance on important governing decisions and protect the ruling dynasty. Ancestor worship paved the way for how roles and duties were defined in Chinese society—filial piety.

The filial piety we're familiar with today evolved from Confucius's take on filial piety. Confucius had reframed the filial responsibilities of ancestor worshipping to focus on filial responsibilities that bring harmony to the family unit. This would then flow forward and create harmony in society. Thus, a template for Chinese social structure was born. There were two ethical principles in Confucius's guide to

---

23. "The History and the Future of the Psychology of Filial Piety: Chinese Norms to Contextualized Personality Construct," *Frontiers in Psychology* volume 10, Issue 100 (2019), https://doi: 10.3389/fpsyg.2019.00100.

Chinese social interaction: "Favouring the Intimate" and "Respecting the Superior."

"Favouring the Intimate" highlights the preferential treatment of one's kin. It also highlights the concept that children can never fully repay their parents for giving them life. Thus, adult children can return the care to their elderly parents by carrying out filial duties such as looking after them in old age and being respectful of their parents.

"Respecting the Superior" highlights the principle of designating the decision-making role to the superior person in a family. This concept views that it is ethical for a superior to make decisions for family members in inferior positions. This means that parents have absolute authority over children and by extension, anyone from the elder generation will have more say over a junior family member. Traditionally, the superior person is the eldest male in the family as represented by the patriarchal view of the emperor's absolute authority.

So, the filial piety we know of today in the twenty-first century stems from the combination of these two ethical principles along with how many Chinese households looked in the nineteenth and twentieth centuries. Many elderly folks lived with their married children, usually the eldest son. They relied on him, his wife, and their grandchildren to provide them with physical, emotional, and financial support. Daughters who would usually look after her parents would shift her priority to her in-laws once married. There's still an expectation of obedience and submission from junior family members reminiscent of Chinese imperial times, especially for daughters-in-law.

How Filial Piety Affects the Adult Child

In our modern world, expectations of fulfilling filial piety can be harmful. The impact of modernisation can be seen in the growing number of women in the workforce plus the growth of expatriates and immigrants. To expect filial piety to be fulfilled in this context can inhibit one's independence and subconsciously direct adult children to sacrifice their personal desires and interests.

Ironically, this goes against what many parents want for their children: a better life than theirs. One way for our children to have a better life is to help them achieve their desires. But if our children are expected to uphold filial piety, how can they achieve their desires and be truly happy?

Within the context of confinement practice, if our mothers, aunts, and grandmothers found the strict traditional ways constricting, uncomfortable, and impractical for a working woman, it would make sense to want to help the next generation of moms have a better experience. But this doesn't always happen because of filial piety. Because of how ingrained this principle is, it's not easy to just *Hakuna Matata* or "put the past behind you." They probably won't be able to really explain why they can't just walk away from this sense of obligation either. This may come as a culture shock to you if you've never been exposed to such principles while growing up.

The same goes for our spouses or partners who are brought up with filial piety. They can feel obliged to respect their mom's wishes for you to follow the confinement practice. Even if it's not in your culture to do so. Thus, they may not voice out their support for you to modernise the confinement month and/ or they might try to convince you to just follow their mom's wishes for now.

Your spouse or partner can also be affected by your decision to want a modern confinement practice and experience a similar guilt for supporting you. They might feel like they must pick a side. That can lead to stress, anger, and/or anxiety for both of you. Arguments could ensue between all parties. You could feel depressed and lonely if your spouse or partner seems like they're siding with your mom or their mom. They could feel like you're disrespecting their relationship with their mom by not wanting to follow what she says. They could also secretly feel shame for not standing up for you in front of their mom because they do want you to have a modern confinement practice but don't know how to please both sides.

It can get messy, but, again, let's focus on what we have control over—*ourselves*, as the new mom. We may not be able to untangle all the chaos, but we can keep our corners organised by managing our expectations and setting boundaries.

We'll start with managing our expectations and then talk about setting boundaries. Why in this order? It's easier to make a list of what you want and don't want. But whether you can really have those things happen is another story. To make our list of boundaries practical, it's more productive to first manage our expectations.

SOMETHING TO THINK ABOUT BEFORE THE EXERCISES IN THIS CHAPTER

The 5 Love Languages by Gary Chapman! I highly recommend everyone in your family and/or confinement support network take the quiz in his book or from the website (5lovelanguages.com/quizzes) to discover what your primary and secondary love languages are.

For the new mom: Knowing your love languages is a powerful way of ticking your emotional boxes during the confinement month and for the rest of your postpartum journey. This can also help you set better expectations and set a main confinement goal because you're able to ask yourself if these are fulfilling your love languages.

For spouses and partners: Knowing their love languages can help you learn how to express gratitude to them during the confinement month.

For moms and MILs: Knowing their love languages can help with the other exercise in this chapter when it comes to crafting a way to tell them about wanting to practice a modern confinement practice.

For other children in the family: Gary Chapman has written a love language book specifically for children and teenagers. Learning their love languages can be helpful in navigating the confinement month and Postpartum Year to help them continue feeling loved, included, seen, and heard.

HOW TO MANAGE EXPECTATIONS FOR THE CONFINEMENT MONTH

Let's KISS: Keep It Super Simple! With only two steps to reframe your expectations of your confinement month, you can repeat this exercise for the rest of the Postpartum Year when needed.

Step 1: Identify Your MAIN GOAL for the Confinement Month

Just one. One goal that you'd like to achieve during the confinement month. Why only one? You've got so much recovery to do, it's practical to only have one goal!

Here are some ideas:

- **Peace:** The focus of this goal is to have as few arguments and little tension as possible!
- **Settle into our growing family:** This goal aims to help you enjoy your plus one into the family! Arguments and tension may occur but since the main goal is to settle into a growing family, you and your spouse or partner may let peace slide from time to time.
- **Have home help:** You might want your mom, MIL, or a hired confinement support person to live with you during the entire confinement month. Or you might want to hire doulas and/or nighttime baby nurses to help on certain days of the week during your confinement month.

Step 2: Create a Plan

Brainstorm by yourself and then include your spouse or partner (if you have one or if they'd like to join in). Set a timer for 10 minutes and scribble away. Refer to your main goal to guide you: *What do you expect your confinement month to be like?*

Write out all the expectations you can think of, then screen each one with the following questions (where applicable and in no particular order). Keep referring to your main goal to guide you.

- Do I/we have the physical space at home to do this?
- Can I/we afford this?
- Can I/we easily buy or borrow things/ingredients to make this happen?
- How will I/we feel if we cannot have this?
- How will I/we feel if we can have this?
- How will my mom and/or MIL likely feel about this?

Sound off with your spouse or partner, or a friend or family member. They might have ideas or further questions that can be the final piece to your puzzle!

Write your refined expectations down as mantras that can help you navigate difficult moments if and when they pop up during the confinement month and Postpartum Year.

With your expectation mantras and main confinement goal in hand, let's work on setting some boundaries for the confinement month. You can write them out in a way that can also serve as a visitor etiquette list. And you can always adapt this for the rest of the Postpartum Year as needed.

HOW TO SET BOUNDARIES FOR THE CONFINEMENT MONTH

We'll make our list based on the following themes while referring to our expectation mantras and main confinement goal. I'll dive into the three main boundaries that are commonly set during the confinement month.

Physical Boundaries

These relate to visitors and physical interactions. These boundaries are set to allow new moms to rest, and to give the growing family space during this tender time. So, the boundaries you list here can also apply to your spouse or partner. It's also to protect the newborn from overwhelming exposure to too many new elements and folks over a short time since they need time to adjust to being outside the womb. Plus, their immune system is still so immature. Examples of physical boundaries related to confinement month and the Postpartum Year are as follows:

- No visitors in our home during the entire confinement month.
- No kissing the baby. Only you and your spouse or partner can kiss the baby.
- Don't ask to carry our baby.
- Knock, and then enter our bedroom only if we say, "Come in," unless there's an emergency.
- We will not serve you or entertain you during this time.
- No sex or any intimate physical touch until I'm ready.
- Do not rearrange our things in these rooms.
- Mom, I'd love to get help with food and chores only. I want to focus on healing and learning how to care for my new baby during this time. If I need more help, I will ask you.

Emotional Boundaries

These relate to unsolicited advice and comments, and criticisms. Setting emotional boundaries aims to protect your and your partner or spouse's feelings and thoughts—your mental and emotional health. Examples of emotional boundaries related to confinement month and the Postpartum Year are as follows:

- We will not tolerate discussions about body shape, size, weight, and appearances during this time.
- If you have nothing nice to say, say nothing.
- Please do not make comments about our baby's appearance and size.
- Mom, *sensei* said I'm not supposed to feel too much emotional stress but I'm starting to feel very upset now. I'd like to rest for a bit.

Technology Boundaries

Social media, phones, computers, TV, Internet, shows, and movies! Of course, social media is a big contentious topic in our twenty-first century. Many of us may not want pictures of us just having given birth or of our new baby plastered on someone's social media post when we're not ready to share anything. We also may not want to watch certain shows or deal with certain phone calls or texts during the confinement month that could annoy or stress us out. Examples of technological boundaries related to confinement month and the Postpartum Year are as follows:

- No posting any of our pictures on social media. No sharing of our photos to anyone else. These photos are only for you to view.
- Please block out our baby's face with an emoji or blur it out before posting any pictures with our baby in it.

- No emotional Disney movies for the month! No true crime TV shows either, especially those relating to children.
- I'll be offline from social media during my confinement month.

Other Boundaries

A few other themes you can use when setting boundaries include the following:

- **Time boundaries:** How you spend your time during the confinement month and Postpartum Year.
- **Material and Financial boundaries:** How you spend your money and other assets during the confinement month and Postpartum Year.
- **Spiritual and Religious boundaries:** How you worship or carry out spiritual activities during the confinement month and Postpartum Year.
- **Non-negotiable boundaries:** These boundaries are deal breakers. Things can get very sensitive for everyone. Set these where necessary and refer to the dynamics in your family. These boundaries include vaccination status, smoking, pets, guns, or others that you consider must-haves to feel safe.

There's also a unique challenge when it comes to Asian moms and MILs: how to tell them you want to have a modern confinement practice!

Remember we talked about how emotional this is rather than logical. So, the recommendations I'm offering below touch on the emotional side for you and your mom and/or MIL. I personally wouldn't bring up science, data, and medical talk. Have your main confinement goal, expectations, and list of boundaries ready too, including a copy for mom and/or MIL. Remember to reword the list you have for them so that they feel included and respected!

There are two parts to getting them on board. First, breaking the news of you wanting to do confinement your way and/or by yourself. Second, telling them how they're still playing a part in your confinement practice and beyond. This way, they can still flex their elderly wisdom when you're ready for it!

Breaking the News

Keep this part short and sweet. Dragging out your explanation is likely to convolute things rather than simplify. Good reasons that can hold up against all sorts of guilt-tripping and negotiations might include:

- We want our own space to grow into our new family of [insert new number]
- I want my spouse or partner to be my confinement support person
- My spouse or partner wants to be my confinement support person
- We want to do confinement by ourselves due to all the health concerns nowadays

But let's pave the way for them in a gentler and inclusive way. This can be before or during your pregnancy.

- Take your mom/MIL out for a meal or cook for her. Food is the love language of many Asian moms. After that, try starting a conversation with your elders about their experience with confinement and/or their birth story(ies). Take this chance to ask them how they felt during their confinement. Goodness knows the older generation and Asian culture avoid talking about emotions, but this is a chance to bond over a very intimate ritual and tradition.

- Plan the confinement month together! Even if you're planning to do your confinement month by yourself and/or your partner or spouse. This is also a great time to go through your main confinement goal, expectations, and list of boundaries. And to show your mom and/or MIL that you have a solid confinement plan for the month! If they don't like certain things about your plan, you can bring in the 100-day or Fourth Trimester confinement plan (see below) and "let them" run things for a little time after your primary confinement month.

- Prepare for your confinement together! Your mom and/or MIL can help with preparing meals to freeze, marinate things in advance, and bottle sauces. Your spouse or partner can also learn how to cook certain confinement meals from your mom and/or MIL during the pregnancy. This is a wonderful way of proving that your spouse or partner is a capable cook!

The 100-Day or Fourth Trimester Confinement Plan

In this confinement plan, you'll do the first 30 days of confinement by yourself and/or with your spouse or partner or confinement support person of your choice. Then your mom and/or MIL can help you during the rest of the 70 days or for the rest of the Fourth Trimester by supporting you with more confinement foods, helping with baby and other kids if you have them, helping you with chores, and whatever else you might need. The 100-day confinement plan is a good way to coincide with your baby's 100th day celebration (see chapter 10). This plan is also useful for births that need longer recovery time like C-sections or a difficult/traumatic birth.

If having your mom and/or MIL stay with you for 70 days or the rest of the Fourth Trimester is too long for you, then shorten that to however long you feel is best for you. Remember, the focus is on you and what benefits you the most!

> *Note to spouses whose mom/family member (FM) will be the confinement support person:* You must decide whether you will intervene if mom/FM oversteps the boundaries that are set up!

I had my mom come stay with us for my confinement month after having my first baby. While it was helpful, it was also stressful, through no fault of my mom's. It was just the dynamics in our home with three headstrong personalities! So, for our second baby, my husband and I decided to do confinement by ourselves. He was my confinement support person, so he learned to prepare all my confinement food, teas, and soups.

He took care of the house and our toddler while I rested and focused on our new baby. We were also able to hire a cleaning person to help 1–2 times a week with chores for the month. This was a game-changer and I'm thankful we were financially able to afford it. I loved this approach so much more because I felt we were able to grow into our family of four at our own pace and in our own space.

My mom came over after my husband finished his paternity leave of 30 days (he took extra leave to make sure he could care for me for the entire 30 days). She still cooked some confinement foods and teas for me, which was wonderful for her. And my husband and I gladly "let her" take over the kitchen.

Now that you're armed with background knowledge about the Postpartum Year and the Chinese postpartum confinement practice and have an idea about how to compromise and communicate with your mother or mother-in-law about your confinement wishes, let's get into the practical side of things: how to apply these practices and how to plan your modern confinement practice!

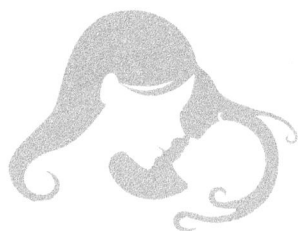

Section 2

The Modern Confinement

Chapter 4

How to Use This Section

Section 2 is written in a way that you can digest small pieces and pick up where you left off without having to go back and reread too much. I wrote this book the way a busy mom tackles everyday tasks: in bite-sized chunks and with questions to guide me!

Once again, I remind you that this book is not a medical textbook and all the recommendations in the following chapters do not substitute for medical advice from your health practitioners. If you have doubts on whether you can or should follow suggestions in this book, please discuss them with your health practitioner. I always encourage this in every chapter.

Most important, you can always adapt my recommendations to suit your unique situation and needs.

The modern confinement chapters (the kitchen; bathroom; bedroom, living room, and outdoors chapters) have the following structure amended to each chapter. Here's what you'll learn in each section:

TRADITIONAL PRINCIPLES

Although I've written about TCM concepts in a nutshell in chapter 1, I've summarised some of the TCM approaches to the confinement practices specific to each chapter. This is also so you can understand the traditional and cultural basis of my modern confinement recommendations. And you don't have to flip back and forth to chapter 1 too! Dr. Kim, a licensed acupuncturist and TCM practitioner, has also kindly shared her wealth of knowledge and expertise in TCM postpartum care, so I've included her input in this section.

POSSIBLE ANCIENT ORIGINS

Here, I discuss possible reasons our ancestors practiced postpartum recovery the way they did and why they viewed things in a certain way. This section is based on my cultural background growing up in Malaysia as a Chinese ethnic female, anecdotes passed on to me by my family and community, and my medical background.

MODERN RECOMMENDATIONS

This is where I bring my medical knowledge and experience and share input from a family medicine specialist (Dr. Pey Shyan, a fellow Malaysian!) about the recovery time during the Postpartum Year from the modern medical perspective. This section combined with the TCM principles section make up the foundation of my modern confinement concept. I'm bridging both worlds toward a practice that is comfortable for the modern mom yet fulfills a connection to Chinese heritage and tradition.

THE MODERN CONFINEMENT APPROACH

The suggestions I make here are based on my personal experiences of practising confinement twice, advice from my mother and aunt, input from my health professional colleagues, and current medical guidelines on postpartum care and other medical conditions. I include options for a traditional approach to the confinement practice so that you've got a guide for going full traditional if you'd like to!

THE BARE NECESSITIES

For busy moms or those of us who can't get the help we need to follow a full confinement practice, there's recommendations in this section in each chapter for the most basic things you can do to reap some benefits of a confinement month. It's important for some of us to partake even in the smallest possible way because of how close we are to our heritage, so this section helps us fulfill that and adapts a basic confinement month into our busy lives.

KEY THINGS TO REMEMBER

Naturally, I've got a summary of important take-away information for each chapter to reinforce the main points.

NOTE TO THE CONFINEMENT SUPPORT PERSON

This section guides spouses, partners, family members, and friends of the new mom on navigating this vulnerable time.

The goal of the confinement support person is to help you have a successful confinement month.

A successful confinement month means sticking to your confinement plan as closely as possible. This means having your meals prepared for you so that you'll eat well and on time, chores taken care of, and help with your baby so that you can focus on resting and sleeping. It's also helpful to get some support in adhering to practices you've chosen to follow especially when it gets difficult. For example, if you've chosen to not wash your hair for 2 weeks but your scalp is itching after a week, your support person can help you stick to your plan by distracting you or being your sounding board for complaints of feeling gross.

So, to increase your support person's confidence in helping you through a successful modern confinement month, I've also included tips on what they might encounter from you and themselves during this time.

Now for the best part: the following chapters can be read in any order that suits your fancy! I've categorised them according to common areas in our homes because it's been easier to think of confinement prep based on where we usually spend our time doing certain activities. It's all about functional organisation rather than what looks pretty!

Chapter 5

The Kitchen

Food and Beverages

How and what we nourish our postpartum bodies with is important, regardless of whether we're following a modern or traditional diet. In fact, having a balanced diet is the best thing we can give our bodies. This is where my modern confinement recommendations come into play.

First, let me give you an overview of what TCM and modern medical advice have to say about postpartum nutrition.

TRADITIONAL PRINCIPLES

"Food is medicine. What we consume helps replenish vital substances with nutrients (such as high caloric and protein foods) to promote healing and induce lactation."

–Dr. Eun Kim, D.C.; L.Ac

The TCM approach to postpartum nutrition generally recommends "hot and warm" ("Yang") food and beverages for all dishes, drinks, and soups to restore maternal health and prevent future diseases. This diet aids in restoring our internal balance and strength and assists our body in compensating for the birth-related blood loss. A "Yang" diet also increases lactation and reduces the risk of developing blood clots. Most importantly, this diet prevents and expels Wind from building up in our body. Recall that Wind is a common and recurring enemy of good health and recovery in TCM. "Hot and warm" includes the temperature of the food and drinks, and also ingredients that are "hot/warm" in nature. Therefore, the opposite also exists. There are "Yin" or "cold/cooling" foods and beverages, as well as neutral ones.

For general reference, here are some examples of cooling foods and warm foods. I've adapted Eu Yan Sang's food list[24] and my mother's recommendations, so these ingredients are a good starting point for reference. However, I'd recommend referring to your TCM provider to be sure about the nature of foods you're planning to consume during your confinement month. The list below does not include many other ingredients also available from your local grocery stores.

"Yin" "Cold/Cooling" Foods

- **Fruits:** apples, bananas, oranges, pears, strawberries, watermelon, mangoes
- **Vegetables:** alfalfa sprouts, asparagus, bitter gourd, celery, cucumber, eggplant, green leafy vegetables, mushrooms, spinach, lettuce, cauliflower
- **Grains, legumes & seeds:** barley, mung bean, soybean, tofu, wheat bran, whole wheat
- **Meat, seafood & dairy:** clam, cheese, chicken egg, crab, yoghurt

---

24. "TCM Basics–Food," Eu Yan Sang, https://www.euyansang.com.sg/en/tcm -basics-%E2%80%93-food/eystcmoverview4.html.

- **Condiments & beverages:** chrysanthemum tea, green tea, peppermint tea, salt, sesame oil, soya sauce

"Yang" "Hot/Warming" Ingredients

- **Fruits:** apricot, cherry, coconut flesh, raspberry
- **Vegetables:** chives, leek, onion, pumpkin, squash
- **Grains, legumes & seeds:** chestnut, glutinous rice, pine nut, walnut, pistachio
- **Meat, seafood & dairy:** butter, chicken, eel, ham, lamb, mussels, prawns, sea cucumber
- **Condiments & beverages:** basil, black pepper, brown sugar, chilli, cinnamon, clove, coffee, cumin, fennel seed, garlic, ginger, rosemary, vinegar, wine

Neutral Foods and Beverages

- **Fruits:** figs, goji berries, grapes, olives, papaya, plums, lemons
- **Vegetables:** black fungus, carrot, Chinese cabbage, corn, potato, sweet potato, turnip, white fungus
- **Grains, legumes & seeds:** almond, kidney beans, peanut, rye, sunflower seed, white rice
- **Meat, seafood & dairy:** abalone, beef, cow's milk, duck, fish, oyster, pork, scallop
- **Condiments & beverages:** peanut oil, honey, rock sugar, white sugar

POSSIBLE ANCIENT ORIGINS

Back in the olden days, it made sense to only serve hot foods, soups, and drinks to a new mother during her recovery month.

Why? This was the best way to ensure that everything was cooked properly and that the water used for teas and soups was clean! Otherwise, the new mother would have been at risk of catching a stomach bug and becoming seriously ill from improperly cooked food or dirty water. Unlike in our modern world, our ancestors didn't always have access to clean water, nor could they always easily boil water at home. And they definitely didn't have the technology to easily produce water filters or build water sanitation plants.

MODERN RECOMMENDATIONS

Mothers are encouraged to eat a balanced diet with enough protein, carbohydrates, and calcium, as well as have adequate hydration. A healthy balanced diet without supplements in the confinement period is usually sufficient to provide us with the nutrients we need, unless we've got anaemia or calcium deficiency. However, for us moms who have complications during pregnancy and after giving birth, we might need to customise our postpartum diet according to the condition. For example, mothers who experience significant blood loss during delivery may need to increase their iron intake during the Postpartum Year.

It's always best to **consult with your health providers** about any conditions you might have and discuss management options. Please also discuss your desire to use herbs and/or complementary therapies!

Limiting the intake of fresh fruit/vegetables (due to the philosophy that many of these ingredients are "cold" in nature) may bring more harm than good since important sources of fibre have been removed from the diet. There's also no current scientific evidence to support avoiding cold fluids in the Postpartum Year. Therefore, from a modern perspective, there's no need to avoid fruits or vegetables that are deemed "cold" in nature.

"As a family medicine doctor, we usually advise mothers to have a healthy and balanced diet. We do not encourage women to avoid certain 'pan-tang'/banned foods, as these are usually not evidence based and it is more of a cultural thing that has been passed down through generations."

—Dr. Pey Shyan, MBBS (Honours)

THE MODERN CONFINEMENT APPROACH

Use the modern amenities we have today,
To make your confinement month easier,
Enjoy your warm confinement food and beverages,
From any food culture you desire!

I'll only be sharing a few of my personal recipes in this chapter because there are many Chinese confinement recipe books and websites. I encourage you to refer to those recipes because those books have been written specifically as cookbooks by women who are very familiar with Chinese herbs and ingredients. My recipes are based on the food my mom cooked for me during my confinement with ingredients that are more readily available in Western grocery stores.

My mom used *The Chinese Pregnancy and Confinement Cookbook* by Ng Siong Mui for her confinement and she passed it down to me. I love this book because it's written by a Singaporean Chinese ("Malaysia's cousin across the Strait" as I like to say) so the concepts and traditions are very similar to the Malaysian Chinese. While our ancestors mainly hailed from South China, many Chinese traditions and customs have evolved over the generations to become unique to the Malaysian Chinese.

Therefore, instead of lots of recipes in this chapter, we'll focus on the functional part of confinement: the preparation of confinement meals.

MY FAVOURITE CONFINEMENT RECIPE RESOURCES

- *The Chinese Pregnancy and Confinement Cookbook* by Ng Siong Mui
- *The First Forty Days: The Essential Art of Nourishing the New Mother* by Heng Ou
- *The Chinese Postpartum Diet* series by the website "The Woks of Life: A Culinary Genealogy" (thewoksoflife.com/chinese-postpartum-diet)
- *Nourishment from Within: A Confinement Cookbook* by Thomson Medical (published by Thomson Medical, a Singaporean hospital)

How to Prepare Food and Beverages for a Comfortable Confinement Month

Food & Beverage Preparation and Storage

Freezing: Yes! You can freeze your ingredients, cooked meals, and uncooked meals! This is a wonderful advantage we have over our ancestors and rest assured, my TCM collaborators have given the green light to prepare your food ahead of time. Bear in mind that most homemade foods are usually good for 3 months frozen to maintain freshness upon defrosting and reheating. So, go ahead and prepare up to 3 months ahead! This will give you and/or your support person(s) time to slowly stock up food for your confinement month. However, this might mean needing more freezer space than you might have in your regular fridge.

TIP FOR SAVING MONEY AND SPACE

I recommend looking into getting an extra freezer to store your stock. Best search for secondhand freezers and something not too large in case you don't plan to use the freezer after your confinement month. You'd rest easy knowing you didn't spend a ton of money on a brand-new freezer and can just sell it off again after you're done!

You can prepare your meals and drinks in the following manner:

Teas: Some teas you can purchase in tea bags and some you'd like to brew on your own. With specialty confinement teas, many Chinese herbal shops have powdered preparations of the confinement herbs which can easily be made into a hot tea beverage. Or if you'd like to brew your own, you can boil the tea in advance, cool it down, then freeze it. Just make sure you use freezer-friendly bottles! However, if you're using whole herbs prescribed by your TCM practitioner, these are usually best boiled on the day you intend to consume them, unless directed otherwise by your TCM specialist.

See the appendix of this book for my favourite homemade tea recipe: Red Dates Ginger Tea.

Broths/soups: Like teas, you can prepare these in advance! Even better, you can boil concentrated broths to save storage space. Just remember to dilute them when you use them! Bone broths are the best and these make wonderful soup bases for many confinement meals. Where possible, ask for bones (sometimes called soup bones, broth bones, marrow, chicken carcass, pork shoulder bones, beef leg bones) from your local butcher and the meats section of your closest supermarket. These "spare parts" are easily found in many Asian countries and in some Asian grocers, but in a Western neighbourhood, best ask for these parts wherever you can because it's not common that many people want them! Worst case, you can order bone broth powders from specialty shops.

Pre-marinate uncooked meals: You might prefer cooking some meals fresh, like stir-fries with meats, because the meat will be more tender unlike heating up pre-cooked meats. In this case, marinate your ingredients and store them in the freezer immediately after. It'll take time for things to freeze so your food will have sat in the marinade for a good amount of time to absorb the flavour. I prefer to separate the vegetables and meats because they'll cook at different speeds once thawed, but if you don't mind them being cooked together, just throw them all in a marinade and freeze them together!

Cooked meals: Some things can be cooked in advance, such as casseroles and stews. I love rice porridge (a.k.a., congee) so I've frozen batches of cooked porridge with success. You can cook these meals to your taste buds' desires and just freeze them once cooled.

Reheating Stored Food and Beverages

While confinement meals are usually prepared fresh and served immediately, it may not be convenient for us with our modern commitments to do this every day, for 3 or more dishes, for an entire month.

Here are some tips for reheating your meals, soups, and teas without compromising the nutrition:

Stovetop/Ovens: The recommended reheating method is using the stovetop or oven. Why? This method is gentler on the food than the microwave since we can control the heat more easily.

Microwave "Go low and slow": Don't nuke your food on high! It's too easy to do this with our microwaves. Instead, dial down the microwave power and heat it up over a few minutes. I use this method often with success. This applies to teas and soups too.

Steaming: Food steamers are wonderful for reheating cooked meals or cooking prepared meals. If you don't have a food steaming appliance, steaming food over boiling water in a wok covered with a large lid will do. I use the wok method since it's the most common way of steaming food back home in Malaysia. You'd need something to elevate your meals from the water in the wok such as a food steaming basket. You can use this to reheat teas and soups too.

Beverage heater: If you have any kind of drink warming appliance, that'll work nicely for heating up your stored teas. Otherwise, you can reheat your teas in a kettle (electric or stove works nicely), the microwave, or by steaming. Sometimes, I use my kid's bottle warmer to heat up my teas—just because the appliance is always accessible and produces the same results as heating my teas up in any other way!

Sample Menus

Here are some meal category suggestions to get your creative juices flowing when planning your confinement menu! I've adapted this from the previously mentioned confinement and pregnancy cookbook by Ng Siong Mui.[25]

This is a good opportunity to have fun with your partner, spouse, or support person and merge your culinary cultures and family traditions! If in doubt whether an ingredient is "Yin," "Yang," or neutral in nature, consult your local TCM practitioner, pharmacist, or herbalist.

Breakfast: Something easy to prepare during your likely sleep-deprived mornings or a meal that can be prepared in a slow cooker the night before will be a very convenient breakfast dish. Hydration first thing in the morning after a long night is also very important.

- Rice porridge/congee with ginger, veggie, and meat

---

25. Ng Siong Mui, *The Chinese Pregnancy & Confinement Cookbook* (Singapore: Landmark Books, 1990)

- Confinement tea or other teas
- Sandwiches
- Water (room temperature or warm)

Lunch: This is a good time to prepare heartier foods and also dinner meals. Why? It's likely you'll have some energy to do more cooking before the late afternoon stupor and early evening anxiety hits. If possible, cook for dinner too.

- Fried rice
- Noodles
- Wraps
- Stir-fries
- Soups

Dinner: I personally detest preparing dinner. Even before I had kids! Something about having to put in more effort after a long day (not to mention cleaning up after!) for a meal to wind down with seems counterproductive. So, batch cooked pre-prepared meals that are easy to oven, microwave, or reheat on the stove will be extremely helpful for dinners.

- Stews
- Casseroles

Snack: Honestly, any of the meals above can be treated as a snack if you have a small portion. During the confinement month, it's important to eat whenever you're hungry because your body is doing so much work to recover while producing milk (for breastfeeding moms) and keeping up with energy needs for day-to-day functioning. Here are some snack ideas:

- Lactation cookies (if you need to boost breastmilk production—but beware of eating too many at once! Breast engorgement can occur if you respond very well to the ingredients in lactation cookies)
- Veggies
- Nuts
- Biscuits and Cookies
- Soups

Beverages: Ones you can switch up during the month so you don't get too bored of the same thing:

- Red dates and ginger tea
- Prune juice or pear juice at room temperature or warmed if that suits your taste—to help alleviate constipation
- Teas that are "Yang" in nature

Recommendations of other daily intake items

- Prenatal vitamins
- Room temperature or warm water
- Red dates and ginger tea
- Stool softeners
- More fruits and veggies to prevent constipation if not using stool softeners. Make sure to hydrate often to avoid having the fibre consolidate and cause or worsen constipation!

Services for Confinement Meals and Ingredients

I don't provide country-specific services in this section because you, dear reader, may hail from different parts of the world. What I'll provide here are keywords and concepts that you can search for in your country that are related to the confinement month.

Food Services: You might be able to find a specialty confinement food delivery service that covers your full month of confinement meals. Such services might use the following words:

- Confinement food
- Postpartum meals
- Confinement meals

Otherwise, consider meal delivery services where you can choose the type of meals you get. You can always add confinement friendly ingredients to these recipes and remove non-recommended ingredients. The best part is the food doesn't go to waste because other members of your family can use the ingredients that are left out!

Confinement Agencies: If you're able to access confinement agencies in your area, many of them offer confinement support persons for hire for the entire month! This person, usually an older lady, will cook all your confinement meals and help with the baby too. Some can stay over in your home for the month if that suits everyone. However, the cost might not work out for everyone and some of us may not like a complete stranger to come tell us what to do (and what NOT to do) for a whole month!

Traditional Chinese Medicine clinics and herbal shops: One of the easiest things to do to save money is to grab a month's worth of confinement herbs from your trusted TCM herbal shop. I'd recommend seeing a TCM specialist so that you can discuss your needs prior to being prescribed the herbs. Some of us may not want to breastfeed and the specialist can prescribe herbs that don't stimulate lactation. I wanted to give breastfeeding a try, so the specialist I saw made sure to include lactation boosting herbs in my prescription. Some of these clinics and shops may be able to give you herbal preparations in powder/granule form, which can easily be made into a pot of tea to be taken throughout the day or in one go; whichever suits your fancy! Make sure the tea is always warm though.

Takeout & Substitutes

As much as we love fast food, it's recommended to satisfy this craving after the confinement month. It's best to stick to foods prepared with less processed ingredients so that our bodies can reap the most nutrition as we heal. BUT! If the craving is just too intense, go for it! I've had a few fast food meals during my confinement month to satisfy some deep cravings for an American-style juicy burger.

Home cooked meals are always recommended during confinement because we're in control of most of the ingredients we use. Plus, freshly cooked meals are considered healthier than takeout. However, if you're short of time, energy, or have a restaurant you love and trust, by all means, order takeout! Even better if they can accommodate requests for substituting or removing non-recommended ingredients.

CHALLENGES OF PREPARING FOOD DURING YOUR CONFINEMENT PERIOD

It takes a lot of effort to prepare fresh, home-cooked meals in our modern lives. Why? Access to fresh and good quality ingredients can be limited depending on where you live. Time can be limited due to long work hours and long commuting times if your partner, spouse, or support person doesn't have parental leave—and even if they're working from home! So, if and when you need to order takeout, please do so.

Got a Western dish you love? Yes, please cook those! Again, substitute or remove the non-recommended ingredients and enjoy your favourite meal.

Vegetarians and vegans! Substitute meats with relevant plant proteins (lentils, chickpeas, bean curd, quinoa, oats, nuts, sweet potato, broccoli, spinach). Please engage your vegan friends and communities, and TCM health providers for ideas on vegan ingredients that are confinement friendly.

It's challenging enough to manage your healing, a new baby, your family and home, plus the roller-coaster of emotions during your first month at home after childbirth. At the very least, let's give our taste buds a wonderful confinement experience and be less strict about sticking ONLY to Chinese confinement foods!

IMPORTANT TIPS!

HYDRATE, HYDRATE, HYDRATE: It is recommended to increase fluid intake (water more than anything else, please!) especially if breastfeeding since most women feel quite thirsty when feeding their baby. Hydration also helps the body recover well and reduces postpartum swelling.

Make sure that you don't skip meals or go for long periods without eating. Try to eat small, nutritious snacks throughout the day to maintain energy levels.

THE BARE NECESSITIES

- Tea bags (Green tea, Corn silk tea)
- Most basic ingredients to use in cooking, soups, and teas:
  » Ginger
  » Red dates/jujube
  » Goji berries/keiji
  » Protein and iron-laden ingredients
- Consume everything warm or at room temperature
- Eat a balanced diet and hydrate often

KEY THINGS TO REMEMBER

- Avoid all cold temperature foods, drinks, and soups!
- Consume everything warm or at room temperature.
- Always choose the easiest recipes, preparation methods, and cooking methods that suit your needs.

- Boil your teas, water, and soups and allow them to cool to room temperature instead of letting something cold come to room temperature.

MAKING THE CASE FOR PREPARING DRINKS WITH BOILING WATER IN OUR MODERN ERA

Pathogens, microbes, bacteria, spores, and bugs still exist in our ingredients and produce, either naturally or introduced during production. Just because we have factories to mass produce food and goods that are usually pretty well managed from a public health perspective, and medicine to cure many ailments, doesn't mean we should be complacent with our food and beverage preparation at home.

Preparing teas, formula for babies, and powdered drinks for ourselves with boiling water helps kill dormant spores, eggs, and such in the powder. Babies' immune system and gastrointestinal immune environment are still weak at such a tender age, so ensuring their formulas are well-prepared is very important in preventing food-borne illnesses. Similarly, for us new moms, the body is weakened after birth so preventive measures to avoid exposure to illness is always helpful.

Stir the mixture or let your tea bags sit in boiling water for 5 minutes before adding water to cool it down. In the case of soups, reheating it on the stove till it's boiling is better than in the microwave. Let cool to a comfortable warmth for consumption.

Why 5 minutes? This is the recommended time frame for sterilising baby bottles, teats, caps, and pacifiers in boiling water. So, I adapted this time frame for ease of remembering how long to let your beverage preparations brew in the boiling water.

NOTE FOR THE CONFINEMENT SUPPORT PERSON

- Organise a confinement herbal package or food service: There are many confinement food services or herbal packages to make things easy for you and the new mom for the month. Try searching online using keywords like "confinement package, confinement herbs, confinement service, confinement food, and confinement meals."

- To cut down on work for you if you've got to feed a larger family, choose recipes with the new mom that everyone can enjoy. Otherwise, use the same ingredients to whip up a slightly different dish for yourself and the others. Alternatively, if the new mom doesn't mind and won't feel left out, just order pizza for yourselves! I didn't crave much greasy food during my confinement month, so I absolutely encouraged my husband to order pizza or burgers for himself and our toddler whenever he felt like it.

- Clean up the kitchen as you cook. It's common sense that this cuts down the clean-up work after but it's not easy to stick to it every time you're in the kitchen. If it gets overwhelming at times, ask others to help you clean and/or cook. Although you're supporting the new mom, you absolutely need help from time to time too! Always ask for help and never feel afraid to ask for that help!

There! You've done it. You've gone through the largest part of a confinement month, the food preparations!

The next few practices are a lot easier to prepare and plan for, so let's leave the kitchen for now and head into the bathroom.

Chapter 6

The Bathroom

Hygiene Practices

We've all come across some version of this phrase, "Cleanliness is next to godliness." Well, cleanliness is also next to good health. Labour and childbirth are such a raw and messy physical and emotional experience. The recovery period itself can also make us feel grimy, on top of how hot or cold the weather gets during that time! So, to help our bodies recover, having good hygiene does matter. Clean wounds mean better healing and less risk of infection. And feeling clean does wonders for our mental health.

But bear in mind that we've got good bacteria on our skin, in our mouth, nose, and gut, and even in our vagina. We need these to thrive so that they can prevent the "bad bugs," the microscopic bugs (viruses, mold/fungus, parasites, and so on) that don't benefit us or can cause us harm, from overwhelming our bodies. So, everything in moderation, please! We don't have to go overboard with hygiene.

Now, let's look at what TCM and modern medical advice have to say about postpartum hygiene practices.

TRADITIONAL PRINCIPLES

"Decrease the number of showers as being wet exposes the body to cold air which can increase chances of illness."

—Dr. Eun Kim, D.C.; L.Ac

As described in chapter 2, TCM principles state that during childbirth new mothers lose a lot of "heat" through blood loss. Blood is viewed as "hot" in nature. Therefore, avoiding hair washing, showers, and baths during the confinement period is to avoid exposure to the "cold" (related to wind and water), which prevents the build-up of Wind in the body. This practice aids in maintaining body warmth during the recovery period, which is essential in rejuvenating mom's health and vitality.

POSSIBLE ANCIENT ORIGINS

Many fatal and debilitating health-related conditions in olden times had a lot to do with poor access to clean water or contamination of water sources. This still exists in underdeveloped nations, and we sometimes see this in first world nations after a natural disaster. So, it made sense for our ancestors to avoid exposure to dirty water and reduce the risk of the new mother getting sick from waterborne diseases. Once again, not everyone back in the day had the means to have clean and boiled water every day. It seemed easier to just not bathe and wash their hair during the entire recovery month.

MODERN RECOMMENDATIONS

Definitely take that shower and wash your hair whenever you want! But baths? Here are a few things to consider when deciding whether a bath is suitable.

1. **Wounds and stitches:** Do you have perineal stitches due to tears during birth? C-section surgical stitches? The general advice for wound care with stitches is to keep the area dry until the stitches are removed and the wound has healed. Why? The added moisture from immersing a freshly stitched wound in water can cause skin and wound breakdown, delaying healing. When a wound is wet, there's also an increased chance of infection (bugs love to breed in wet and warm spaces!). So, the safest thing to do is to avoid baths in tubs and swimming until scar tissue has formed nicely. Easiest thing to do is to wait till after your postpartum check-up with your health provider.

2. Recall from the postpartum physiology chapter (chapter 2) that **the cervix takes some time to return to pre-pregnancy state (i.e., closed).** Even if you've had a C-section, the cervix will still be dilated to some degree due to the hormones released during labour. There's a theory (and concern) that immersion in water (tubs and swimming pools) could introduce bacteria and other bugs into the uterus via the still open cervix, risking a uterine infection. I suggest you discuss this with your health provider to get the most current recommendations about baths and swimming in the first few weeks postpartum.

3. **Are you able to safely and comfortably get in and out of a tub full of water?** Besides wounds and stitches, this is the next most important question I'd ask myself. It's sore enough to walk around slowly let alone use the toilet for poos and pees. I wince thinking about navigating the bathtub in those delicate first weeks after giving birth. However, if you've gotten advice that you can take a bath, then go for it! Just make sure you have the means to do it safely. Have someone help you in and out of the tub or have your bathroom set up with rails and other anti-slip aids.

The safest and easiest way to get relief in your perineal region and also clean it well is to have a sitz bath! Although it says bath, it's not a full body bath. It's a bath specifically for your perineal region (this is the area between the anus and vaginal openings). This little tub is placed over the toilet bowl and you sit in it. The tub is easily purchased online or in your local pharmacies.

How to Prepare a Sitz Bath

- Always follow the set-up instructions that come with your sitz bath kit. There are many varieties out there, so I'll only give general advice on how to prepare one.
- Prepare your choice of water temperature. Warm water is the common go-to since it's soothing and promotes blood flow to the immersed region. This is good for promoting wound healing and soothing haemorrhoids. If cooler water is more soothing for you, then use that.

- Prepare your choice of bath salts or herbal soaks. Follow the instructions that come with what you've purchased.
- Prepare what you'll need during and after the sitz bath. This includes clean pads and underwear.

Items to have ready to use:
  » Clean pad
  » Clean underwear
  » Witch hazel wet towels or similar (Tucks brand is popular in the United States). Use whatever is recommended and easily available to you in your area
  » Perineal cold packs (if you still need these for soothing perineal stitches)
  » Haemorrhoid creams or wipes. Whatever is recommended by your health provider if you developed haemorrhoids during active labour
  » Numbing or cooling sprays for the perineal region. Again, different countries will have different brands. Look for one easily available in your area that's also approved by your health provider

- If you'd like, you can pee and/or poo first. Then clean the area using a peri bottle or bidet. Use gentle water pressure to avoid inflicting pain on the tender areas.
- After that, set up your sitz bath. Place the tub over the toilet then add the water and salts or herbal soak packets (or however your kit and soaks instruct you).
- Sit in the bath for 10–15 minutes. No more than 20 minutes in one sitting to avoid burning your skin (if using warm water) and over-soaking your stitches, if any.

- General advice is to repeat up to 3 times a day. Check with your health provider how often you can use a sitz bath soak.
- Remember to keep your sitz bath kit and tub clean! Wash with soap and air dry. If you can, let it sit in the sun occasionally for a good dry.

THE MODERN CONFINEMENT APPROACH

Use the modern amenities we have today,
To make your confinement month easier,
Keep your showers warm and quick,
And always get dried and dressed
before you leave the bathroom!

This chapter focuses on answering the question, *How do we compromise on traditional hygiene practices to suit our modern needs?*

Showers, Baths & Hair Washing

I've got a few options here depending on how strict you'd like to follow the confinement hygiene practice.

Modern

- Shower and wash your hair whenever you want! Baths depend on the advice from your healthcare provider.
- Other hygiene practices as you please since the fully modern option doesn't follow any confinement rules.

Traditional

- No shower, baths, or hair washing for the entire confinement month.
- Use dry shampoo if your scalp feels itchy.
- Wipe down with a warm towel if you feel uncomfortable but make sure there is no cool air blowing at you when you do this. Dry off completely before stepping out of the bathroom.

Mixed Modern-Traditional

- Showers and hair washing are permitted. No baths.
  - » *"Recommended no baths because of sitting too long in water that doesn't stay warm enough"* (Dr. Eun Kim, D.C.; L.Ac).
- Take quick and warm showers to decrease the time and number of showers during the month.
  - » A personal tip from my mother: My mom prepared a warm ginger water rinse for me to use at the end of my shower as her way of reducing my exposure to Wind since I wanted to shower during the confinement month. It didn't hurt my 2nd degree–tear stitches, so I used this rinse after each shower.
  - » **Mummy Jo's Ginger Rinse:** Dice a handful of fresh peeled ginger. Boil in 2 litres of water on medium-high heat for about 5 minutes. Turn off heat and allow ginger to steep for another 15 minutes. Use as a warm rinse after showers. You can add warm shower water to the rinse if needed. Please test the temperature of the rinse before using.

- No hair washing for the first 2 weeks. I used dry shampoo during this time. When I started washing my hair, I washed it every other day.
  - » *"My compromise was 1–2x/week. Nowadays most women are washing their hair less anyway"* (Dr. Eun Kim, D.C.; L.Ac).
- Whenever you wash your hair, ensure it's completely dry before stepping out of the warm, steamy bathroom. Use a hair dryer! It's thought that air-drying damp hair can bring about headaches and migraines, especially during a vulnerable time such as the confinement month.
- Fully dry yourself as best as possible and get dressed before stepping out of the warm, steamy bathroom.
- Ensure your bathroom is warm and no chilly drafts are present.

SAFETY TIP

Please have some water with you in the bathroom and a place to sit (a chair, a stool, or just a towel on top of the closed toilet seat lid). Taking warm showers and baths and remaining in a warm room while you dry off and get dressed can make you feel dizzy if your blood vessels dilate too much due to the heat. I've faced this issue many times and I find drinking water after I take my shower and while I finish up helps a lot. Having a place to sit helps too because your dilated blood vessels don't have to work so hard to pump blood up to your brain. Also, if you have any complications from pregnancy and birth, or have any limitations that make standing to shower uncomfortable, consider getting a shower chair!

THE BARE NECESSITIES

Stick to short, warm showers regardless of how strict or modern you choose to follow in this section. And always get dressed before you leave the bathroom to maintain warmth in your body!

KEY THINGS TO REMEMBER

- Only use warm water! No washing in cold water for the entire month.
- Get fully dressed and hair fully dried in your steamy, warm bathroom.
- Bring water with you and have a place to sit as you finish up in case the warmth dilates your blood vessels too much and causes you dizziness.

NOTE FOR THE CONFINEMENT SUPPORT PERSON

- Help the new mom dry her hair if she's washing it. Or help her with dry shampoo application and brushing after to help her with hair grooming
- Keep her bathroom with essentials well stocked; does she need more pads/adult diapers, tucks, soaps, and so on?
- Help her prepare and clean up her sitz bath.
- Help her to and from the toilet if she's feeling very sore.
- Ask for help with cleaning the bathroom if needed. Toilet duty isn't desirable but someone's gotta do it! A clean bathroom just makes everyone feel better.

Now that you have ideas on how to design a hygiene practice to suit your needs and wants, let's check out the areas of our home that are usually associated with rest, entertainment, and rejuvenation.

Chapter 7

The Bedroom, Living Room, and Outdoors

Rest and Rejuvenate

Recovery can get boring. Given how busy many of us are in our daily lives, imagine having to go from that to resting all day and night! I mean, we'll be plenty busy with our newborn and other children (if we have them) but repeating the same tasks with these guys for a month would drive anyone up the wall.

Not only that, ever heard of the idiom, "An idle mind is the devil's playground"?

Yep. Resting without doing other healthy activities like light exercise and keeping the mind active can allow bad thoughts to seed and take root. But we'll explore more about mental health in the next chapter.

For now, let's dive into some R&R: Rest and Rejuvenate!

Let's start with what TCM and modern medical advice have to say about postpartum rest and exercise.

TRADITIONAL PRINCIPLES

TCM philosophy views pregnancy and childbirth as incredibly taxing on the body, depleting it of "Yang" energy. An imbalance of the "Yin" and "Yang" energy is believed to bring illness. Therefore, bed rest for a month was practiced because resting and avoiding many activities, particularly domestic chores and working, was viewed as important in helping restore the internal balance. Reading, watching TV, or using our mobiles are also discouraged because they are believed to cause problems with eyesight later in life due to unnecessary strain and drying of the eyes.

However, we've come to understand now that resting too long in bed weakens the muscles and reduces our overall strength.

> "Light exercise is recommended to move the Qi and blood, and should not be strenuous to avoid sweating. There's already loss of fluids from birth, so we do not want to further strain the remaining body fluids."
>
> —Dr. Eun Kim, D.C.; L.Ac

POSSIBLE ANCIENT ORIGINS

Without the modern medical care and knowledge we have today, women dying or barely surviving childbirth was very common back in the ancient times. For women who survived, experiencing blood loss was the most common side effect of giving birth. This is tied to low energy. So, it made sense that our female ancestors were prescribed bed rest and avoidance of many activities for the entire month with the aim of rejuvenating the body through resting. But what wasn't as well documented back then was that prolonged rest and avoidance of activities weakened the body instead (because the muscles weren't used over a long period of time).

Reading and engaging in entertainment that could evoke strong emotions were discouraged back in the days because of the TCM philosophy that strong emotions can upset the internal "Yin" and "Yang" balance and because of how many of the Chinese view emotional outbursts unfavourably. (We'll explore more about strong emotions in chapter 8.)

MODERN RECOMMENDATIONS

Rest is always welcomed because, as new moms, we need to regain our energy to tackle the next day. However, bed rest for days or for the entire month is not recommended unless there's a medical reason for it. Why? As mentioned above, prolonged bed rest weakens the muscles due to not using them and this weakens our overall body. Imagine having to run after your other kids after resting in bed for a month! For some moms, we've got to go back to work sooner than we'd like due to poor maternity leave policies. Imagine going back to work after so much bed rest! Our core muscles will undoubtedly not function very well. Sitting and laying down too long also brings the risk of developing blood clots (a.k.a., venous thromboembolic event, VTE).

Just recall the days when you've got a bad cold or a stomach bug. You probably had to lay in bed for a few days to sleep and recover but when you got up and going again, oh how weak you'd gotten! This is why, in modern medical care, we've got our physiotherapists going around in the wards to get patients up and moving as soon as possible. Even after major surgeries! Just changing positions every so often from laying down to sitting, from sitting to standing, and moving to and from the toilet helps us maintain some strength. This helps in postpartum recovery too.

Naturally, only light exercise is recommended while you're healing. A rule of thumb is to only lift things as heavy as your baby for the first 6 to 8 weeks after giving birth! Even better if you have help and only need to lift your newborn and nothing else. This includes after vaginal and C-section births.

"The highest risk of developing a venous thromboembolic event (such as a deep vein thrombosis or pulmonary embolus) is during the first 6 weeks postpartum and hence we encourage women to be as active as their body allows them to be. We encourage daily walks, keep active and to keep well hydrated."

−Dr. Amanda Wee, MBBS, MRMed, MRANZCOG
Obstetrics and Gynaecology Advanced Trainee

"LET'S TALK ABOUT SEX, BABY"

From the ancient aspect of TCM philosophy, refraining from sexual intercourse is advocated because it could endanger and bring bad luck to the family. Some families might still expect the new mother to practice this due to taboos surrounding sex or they simply still follow the ancient beliefs. Sex during this time is also believed to impair the healing of our uterus after giving birth.

Modern medical care advises to avoid sex for the first 6 to 8 weeks after childbirth to allow healing of wounds. Some of us might have perineal tears from vaginal births (and healing time varies based on how severe the tears are!) and some of us must recover from C-sections. Some of us might have other birth-related complications that are scary and require a longer time for physical recovery. The cherry on top is the emotional recovery all of us go through after giving birth. Therefore, many doctors nowadays advise moms to return to sex whenever they feel ready instead of just adhering to the recommended time frame above.

THE MODERN CONFINEMENT APPROACH

My modern confinement R&R philosophies are these:

Growing and birthing life is honourable
yet extremely taxing,
So use this month to get some well-earned rest,
And rejuvenate your spirit,
In whatever way that works for your modern lifestyle!

This chapter focuses on answering the question, *How can we compromise on traditional practices to suit our modern definition of rest and use it with current clinical evidence on postpartum exercise?*

Short answer: We rest when we need to but we have to get up and move every few hours while we're awake. Moving around and keeping active during recovery prevents blood clots from forming in the veins and maintains muscle strength.

Of course, if you have a medical condition or pregnancy-birth complication that doesn't allow you to move around as much as you'd like, take it slowly. As with all other recommendations in this book, these are just guidelines and suggestions that you can adapt to your unique situation and needs.

> **IMPORTANT TIP**
>
> Expect bad days where you feel all the progress you've made to recover some energy and strength has flown out the window. Some days you'll probably even feel you've taken 2 steps back for every step forward. That is normal! You've just brought a new life into this world, and you'll be giving your all to this little one 24/7. BE KIND TO YOURSELF! We'll discuss how to manage setbacks in Chapter 9: Personalising Your Confinement Practice.

Rest

There are many ways we can rest. There's the TCM recommended bed rest, but what we know today has proven that prolonged bed rest deconditions our muscles. So, limit bed rest for sleeping and when you've had a particularly exhausting day or have lots of pain you need to recover from. Just don't stay in bed or on the couch for long periods of time for the entire month unless your doctor has advised you to do so for the safety of your health.

You could also rest by having some quiet time to yourself without the baby, kids, and partner. You could meditate, listen to your favourite music, or watch some TV. This helps you recharge emotionally and physically. Having a baby on you all the time, whether you're breastfeeding or not, can make you feel very touched out. This feeling worsens when we have other children cling to us more than before because they don't fully understand why we're not showering them with the same level of attention as before.

Reclining to rest: Sleeping in recliner chairs or couches, or propping yourself in bed to sleep in a reclined position is okay as long as you're comfortable. I found this most comfortable during the first 2 weeks after my C-section just because it was easier for me to go to the toilet from the couch than from the bed. As my wounds got less painful, I started sleeping flat on the bed to allow my belly to stretch out properly.

Exercise

The goal of exercise during the confinement month is just to prevent rapid muscle strength loss. From the TCM perspective, exercise moves the *Qi* and blood, which aids in recovery. Modern medicine also advocates moving often during the recovery weeks to prevent blood clots from building up and to help the lungs ventilate well.

Walk, walk, walk! Short distances and for a few minutes. Even standing for a bit helps the muscles retain their strength. Walking helps the bowels move too. This also removes gas from the abdomen. Ensuring that your pelvic area has room is important for uterine recovery. A full bladder, being gassy, and constipation impinges on the womb and can sometimes cause pain or discomfort.

To help you get going often, set a timer to use the toilet every 2–3 hours. I found this very useful for ensuring I emptied my bladder often after my C-section. Things remained quite numb for me for a couple of weeks after the surgery due to the nerves being affected by the procedure. Even for vaginal births, sometimes the bladder needs some retraining especially after epidurals. Take this chance to walk around for a bit.

Choose only VERY LIGHT exercises and only lift things as heavy as your baby. TCM philosophy recommends light exercise to avoid sweating because sweating puts a strain on an already fluid-depleted body from giving birth. In both TCM's and modern medicine's body of knowledge, our joints become lax and loose during the pregnancy to allow the baby to grow. This takes time to return to the pre-pregnancy state so very light exercises reduce the risk of injuries caused by these unstable joints.

Avoid bending from the waist if you need to reach for low level items. Always bend from the knee (i.e., squat). I'd recommend completely avoiding any exercises that require you to bend from the waist, such as the forward-fold pose in yoga. It aggravates a C-section wound and it's uncomfortable even for us who've had vaginal births.

Wear a belly binder! This helps hold our abdomen together and gives us the core support we've lost. This is very helpful for us with other kids to tend to. I regretted not wearing one after my first kid. I felt a huge difference in core and back support when wearing this after my second baby. Even my C-section aches were relieved while I was wearing the belt. Please only wear this once your pains and wounds are well-managed. Always ask your midwife, nurse, or doctor when you can start belly binding.

Sex

Straight up, no sex! Let's let momma recover and heal up first, okay?

Frankly, both you and your partner are unlikely to feel frisky during the first 30 days after the birth of your child. There's so much going on for both of you that all your energy will likely be spent on figuring out how to adjust to this new bundle of joy plus managing your own emotions, either as first-time parents or psyching yourself to brave the baby stage all over again.

But cuddles, hugs, and kisses are absolutely encouraged! Unless you feel touched out. Do have a chat to your spouse or partner about what works for you both. And spouse and partners, remember, this month is all about mom so please cater to what she wants and needs for now. It'll absolutely help her recover and rejuvenate in every way: physically, mentally, and emotionally.

Entertainment

If you'd like to follow the TCM recommendation on exposing yourself to fewer strong emotions and prevent drying of the eyes, you can reduce screen time and change your type and theme of entertainment for the month. Reducing screen time can be replaced with audio content such as podcasts and audiobooks. Current studies and modern health recommendations for preserving eye health also include reducing screen time due to the damaging blue light.

Changing the type and theme of entertainment to happier and calmer content can help with evoking more positive emotions that are less likely to provoke strong feelings. Avoid social media where possible because of how toxic it can be even when we try our hardest to curate nice content for our feeds.

Bear in mind that stronger emotions are likely to emerge regardless of how well you try to avoid them. This is because our bodies are going through a lot of hormonal and physical changes after giving birth. See chapter 8 for more information on postpartum moods.

MODERNITY AND 24/7 CONNECTIVITY

The media, our parents and peers, and scientific studies have opined about how being connected to each other and the world all the time can be detrimental to our mental and physical health, and relationships. But can we really disconnect? I ask this question because it's easier for people who have the time, money, and energy to leave work and tech behind. It's realistically not as easy for those of us "mere mortals." Depending on which part of the world you're having your baby in, your financial status, parental leave allowance, and support system, maybe you must keep up with social media, the news, and your emails during your confinement month. Because bills must be paid. Food must be put on the table. Diapers and formulas need to be replenished. So, when deciding on how much screen time to consume during your confinement month, be practical about your needs and your family's needs and current situation.

Outdoors

Yes! Please step out for some fresh air on nice days. Of course, don't go out in the rain or when it's very windy.

If you must go out to public spaces, especially for health visits and other important things, make sure to bundle up and keep warm. Wear long-sleeved tops, long pants, socks, and a scarf to keep the neck warm. This is in line with the TCM philosophy of preserving warmth in the body.

SAFETY TIP

Move as often as possible to decrease risk of forming blood clots in the legs. If you're unable to get up and move, paddle your feet up and down often to engage your calf muscles while resting. Wear compression stockings on top of that!

Keep exercises very light during this month. Only lift things as heavy as your newborn. If you stop to wonder whether you should be doing an exercise, the answer is DON'T DO IT. Chances are you'll be over-exerting yourself. Your body clearly made you stop to think twice!

Ask for help, even if you think it's a silly request but your body says otherwise. I know it's difficult to make this request but you'll benefit from doing less now so that you can do more later! Most important, say "YES, THANK YOU!" whenever help is offered. You'll be doing a lot of heavy lifting, physically, mentally, and emotionally, for the rest of motherhood and parenthood. Learning to say "Yes!" and to ask for help during this time will train you to be more accepting of aid whenever you need it as you traverse motherhood and parenthood.

THE BARE NECESSITIES

- **Exercise:** Walking is enough as exercise.
- **Rest:** Rest when you need to but don't just sit or sleep all day. Get up and move every few hours.
- **Entertainment:** Avoid social media content and platforms that you know can cause you upset. This is protective for your mental health during this important recovery month.

KEY THINGS TO REMEMBER

- Do not lift anything heavier than your baby.
- Wear a belly binder to guard your core if you absolutely need to engage in activities that strongly engage the abdominal muscles.

NOTE FOR THE CONFINEMENT SUPPORT PERSON

- Hold a pamper session for the new mom once a week or whenever you feel she needs one: help her with a simple facial, massage her feet and legs, or give her a manicure and pedicure at home. For spouses and partners, this is a wonderful way to reconnect with your loved one too!
- Offer to take the kids out and/or watch the baby for a few hours so that mom and her spouse or partner can have some personal time together. Or for mom herself to have some "Me Time."
- Have your own routine to recharge and relax during this month. Have a friend you can call on to vent when needed so that you can unload elsewhere and make space to hold your loved one's emotions for the month.

Now that we're done with the modern confinement practices, I invite you to come on a journey with me in the next chapter where I challenge a TCM postpartum philosophy head-on: the practice of avoiding intense emotional states.

Chapter 8

Postpartum Depression and Emotions

CONTENT WARNING:
SUICIDAL THOUGHTS AND
THOUGHTS OF SELF-HARM

If you, or anyone you know, is experiencing thoughts of self-harm or suicide, please reach out to the suicide prevention or crisis hotlines in your country. If you can't think of anyone to call or in a worst-case scenario, call the emergency hotline in your country. Here are some emergency numbers:

- USA, Canada, Mexico, Philippines: 911
- Malaysia: 999
- Singapore: 995 for medical and fire emergencies. 999 for police.
- Australia: 000
- New Zealand: 111
- Germany, France, and any European Union countries: 112
- UK: 999 or 112

My first pregnancy was uncomplicated, but I probably had some level of depression that went unrecognised.

The birth also went well; my baby and I didn't suffer any terrible complications. I had a second-degree tear that was sewn up well and healed wonderfully. My body felt weird after giving birth, but I was mainly okay with that. I knew from my medical background that it'd take time to recover. My body shape and size would also fluctuate for a while before settling into something more regular. And honestly, it would never look the same as before I got pregnant. I just needed to be patient and kind to myself.

My baby was thriving although not sleeping well. That's okay, we were coping. My husband was supportive and my mom came to the United States to help me with my confinement month too. My in-laws were also in town, and they were very understanding and sweet, always making sure my husband and I were ready for any short or long visits, always leaving when we said we needed rest or space.

But although I looked mostly okay on the outside, I was reeling from a roller-coaster of emotions on the inside. Grief. Loss. Happiness. Joy. Guilt. Sadness. Thankfulness. Gratefulness. Love. Doubt. Confusion. Fear.

It's very jarring to feel all these emotions in one go. Yes, all together in one go.

Most worrying to me was this sense of loss. Why did I feel like I'd lost something and had a huge gaping hole in my heart?

As the weeks went by, I felt I was losing my old self. I felt I didn't know who I was anymore. It seemed like all my dreams and ambitions were lost forever because I was now a mother and I should be sacrificing everything for my child just like the women before me did. Like my mother did. I also started beating myself up for experiencing this sense of grief and loss because I really shouldn't be feeling this way. I should be happy, feeling bliss, and cooing at my baby's cuteness, right?

And when I talked about this inner conflict, I usually encountered the question, "Why would you feel like you lost something?" or told (with the best intentions), "You don't have to give up everything for the baby. You're still you." I started feeling crazier, as though I was becoming some dramatic, attention-seeking, ungrateful person. I eventually stopped talking about this uncomfortable feeling of loss on top of other issues I was facing at the time because I got tired of trying to explain something I couldn't understand myself.

This was before I learned about matrescence and what it was (the process of becoming a mother).

Unsurprisingly, I ended up developing full-blown postpartum depression (PPD). I gradually lost my appetite and could only tolerate eating a slice of cheese and drinking milk as my main meals for days. Consequently, my breastmilk supply dropped and my baby couldn't get enough from me. She cried harder and longer than usual. I started feeling more useless, more guilty, and more stressed on top of my grief. It got really bad.

But I was in denial and embarrassed, so I didn't seek professional help immediately. I knew what I was experiencing from a medical perspective but as a "patient"? Yeah, I was a horrible patient. Mainly because I felt like I had failed in managing myself and my emotions. I also started feeling guilty, "Maybe I didn't do my confinement properly, so I developed PPD!" I felt like a bad mom, a bad daughter, a bad wife, and a failure of a person.

One day, I didn't feel safe to be at home alone anymore. I thought to myself, "Ken and Kira will be better off without me. Everyone would be!" Somehow, my logical, medical brain kicked in. In tearful desperation, I rang my psychiatric nurse. I had seen her twice before this but hadn't opened up much to her. But during this call, my floodgates burst open.

I don't remember how, but she managed to calm me down and asked me to get PPD treatment ASAP. And to call my husband immediately! He came home and I asked him to remove all medications from the house. He packed them all up and hid them somewhere.

I also called my OBGYN the same day and he prescribed me antidepressants. I got my meds that afternoon.

My psych nurse saved me from my worst that day. She truly did. It still scares me to think what would've happened if I hadn't called her or if I hadn't met her at all.

Over our next few sessions, she told me I was indeed experiencing grief. She validated that I was feeling a loss for my old self, the me before the jarring, overnight transformation into a first-time mom. She walked me through the 7 stages of grief and, boy, that was a heck of a discovery session!

Looking back, I definitely experienced the many stages of grief. I was in shock and denial in the beginning of my confinement. The first week home after giving birth was a rude awakening into motherhood. I had read about the demands of a newborn but to actually experience it myself was a whole different thing. Yes, I was shaken by how hard everything was. How painful breastfeeding was in the beginning. And I was in denial that I now had to shift my entire life and schedules to centre around the needs of my baby. How dare she upend my routine!

The following week, I started to feel this hole in my gut. This pain was like the feeling I had when I truly realised my grandfather had passed away, a week after his funeral. This pain of loss cut a lot deeper when I started feeling like I'd lost a huge part of myself, as I mentioned above. Then came guilt because why was I feeling this way when I had nothing to worry about? I also felt guilty for being selfish and wanting my old life back. Guilty for feeling like my baby had ended my dreams.

After my confinement, I started feeling angry about everything. I already felt annoyed that I had to defer 4 of my Master of Public Health (MPH) classes and complete them slowly, which meant that I had to graduate later than planned. I was angry at myself for being weak, for thinking that my precious baby was a hindrance to my dreams. I was also angry that I had to defer some dreams of mine and consider letting go of others. Why couldn't I just stay the same person as I was before becoming a mom? Why did it have to be so hard?

I'd say that my PPD hit full-on around the end of my Fourth Trimester. All the guilt, anger, and pain just spiralled into depression once I convinced myself I was alone in this. I felt I was a burden to my husband and friends, I started feeling like my baby and husband would be better off without me, I just wanted to go to sleep and never wake up. But thankfully, I got help before it was too late.

Once I started seeing my psych nurse regularly, I'd walk out of every session feeling validated, feeling better, and more confident in how I'd be able to be the mother I hope to be. It helped very much that although my postpartum grief and loss were unrelated to a miscarriage or stillbirth loss, I was still taken seriously.

I finally felt lighter!

There was also a bubbling excitement from within since I'd been "given" permission to carve a new identity for myself while still having the same dreams and ambitions from before becoming pregnant.

Matrescence is indeed a journey in itself. Looking back, my time in the matrescence period was as long as it needed to be. Knowing what I know now has helped me forgive myself for my "craziness" during that time. And it's helped me accept that it will take time to work things out. Matrescence had a way of reigning me in because whenever I wanted to move forward quicker, the universe would know and give me a right whooping to make me slow down.

I'm still working on myself as I write this book—this chapter. Things are a lot better though! I'm in a better place mentally, emotionally, and socially. And I'm finally starting to enjoy motherhood. Hey, it only took having 2 kids to get me here (about 2 years and 3 months)!

7 STAGES OF GRIEF

The 7 stages of grief evolved from the 5 stages of grief model that was introduced by a Swiss-American Psychologist, Elisabeth Kübler-Ross, in 1969 in a book called *On Death and Dying*.[26]

1. Shock and Denial
2. Pain and Guilt
3. Anger and Bargaining
4. Depression, Reflection, Loneliness
5. The Upward Turn
6. Reconstruction and Working Through
7. Acceptance and Hope

---

26. "Coping with Loss: The 7 Stages of Grief," Shonagh Walker and Sara Mulcahy for HCF, last modified May 2022, https://www.hcf.com.au/health-agenda/body-mind/mental-health/moving-through-grief.

Although grief is described in stages, there's no set start and end stage. A person experiencing grief can process things in any manner, sometimes multiple stages at once. Therefore, grief can be very overwhelming and debilitating at its peak. To explore grief in depth is out of the scope of this book.

Please talk to your loved ones, therapist or counsellor, or health provider if you ever feel like you're feeling a sense of loss you can't quite explain.

I tell my story because I want to share my vulnerability with you. So that you know you're not alone. Especially if you've been brought up to be "not overly emotional" and to believe that "mental health is a Western problem" as viewed in many Asian cultures. It's not easy to find solidarity in such cases.

I hope you'll consider sharing your pain, grief, guilt, happiness, excitement, and everything in between whenever you feel a need to release the pent-up emotions.

Now, although we know how complicated and challenging the path to motherhood and parenthood is, many of us and our elders who were brought up with Chinese culture, and TCM principles tend to view strong emotions as a negative thing. Therefore, all strong emotions should be avoided at all costs during the confinement period!

THE TCM APPROACH TO STRONG EMOTIONS

There are seven main emotions that are considered "internal" causes of disease and illness; anger, joy, sadness, worry, pensiveness (like a sense of longing or something buried deep in your thoughts), fear, and shock. Naturally, there are other "subemotions" under these, such as regret, envy, shame, guilt, frustration, resentment, and hopelessness.

TCM follows the principle that our internal organs belong to the physical-mental-emotional "spheres of influence." That means our mind, body, and emotions exist together as a whole—there's no beginning or end. That's pretty much what a sphere is! All smooth and round, no beginning or end. Because of this, emotional strains can directly "injure" our internal organs.

All we need to understand from this is that any of these emotions can cause disease and illness by "stagnating" your *Qi*. Especially if these emotions are long-lasting, very intense, or both. And remember, when your *Qi* is prevented from flowing and moving, you can fall ill.

An interesting blurb from Maciocia's book *The Foundations of Chinese Medicine: A Comprehensive Text* states, "Emotions become causes of disease when we do not 'possess them' but they 'possess us.'" We'll revisit this blurb later in this chapter.

On the bright side, the "Yin-Yang" concept of balance comes into play here. By default, our internal organs carry positive mental energy. This positive energy turns into negative energy when triggered by emotional strain from our life's circumstances. There's also a chance of emotional imbalance when your internal organs are not in balance with each other. This goes back to the "spheres of influence" concept above!

From the postpartum perspective, the body is viewed as unbalanced after childbirth. So, mitigating emotional strain is even more important to allow the body to recover more efficiently. And to prevent the onset of postpartum-related illnesses, such as postpartum depression.

POSSIBLE ANCIENT ORIGINS FOR EMOTIONAL CONSTRAINT

When you think about it, our hearts race, our faces get flushed, and our blood pressures rise whenever we have strong emotions. Stress puts us on edge or into a "fight or flight" mode while excitement pretty much gets our body going in a similar way. Since TCM sees the postpartum body as out of balance internally, having these extremes of emotions is more harmful than helpful. So, it's best for new moms to maintain emotional stability during the month. This makes complete sense for what our ancestors knew back then.

Plus, many Chinese folks in the past (and today too!) believed that strong emotions were considered unlucky and inappropriate. Why? Unlucky because being emotionally "unstable" was believed to weaken the body and spirit, thus allowing bad luck and bad spirits to attach to you. This was viewed as unfavourable for mom's health and her family's prosperity. Showing emotions was also seen as inappropriate because it meant a lack of self-control and goodness—no one should do that to embarrass themselves and their families!

However, this chapter is wholly dedicated to challenging this cultural view and TCM principle of "controlling your emotions" and "not exposing yourself to strong emotions" during the confinement month. This chapter also challenges the traditional male role where men and fathers are excluded from the confinement practice.

Now that we know the basic philosophy behind emotions, TCM, and Chinese culture, let's talk about postpartum mental health.

MODERN RECOMMENDATIONS FOR POSTPARTUM MENTAL HEALTH

From what we know today about postpartum mental health and matrescence, it can take a while for all our emotions to settle down. Some of us might emerge from this whirlwind of emotions in about 6 months and for some of us it might take longer or shorter. Recall that your body takes 6 to 8 weeks to return to the pre-pregnancy state, hormones included! And many emotional swings you experience during this time are very likely due to your hormones being out of whack.

The baby blues, or postpartum blues, tend to come on within the first week after giving birth and usually resolve by themselves after a couple of weeks or sometimes longer depending on our unique situations. Symptoms of baby blues can feel like depression: sadness, lots of crying, feeling irritated at many things, anxiety, poor sleep, and poor concentration.

Postpartum depression (PPD) is different from the baby blues. To be diagnosed with PPD, most health providers will approach things from a clinical perspective. Meaning, they'll likely use screening questions and follow guidelines set out by the Diagnostic and Statistical Manual of Mental Disorders (DSM). So, the clinical definition of PPD mirrors major depression: Patients must be experiencing a minimum of 5 symptoms and those symptoms must be present for at least 2 weeks. Why is it important to be diagnosed if you do have PPD? It helps all the health providers involved in your care speak the same language. TCM health providers are included because there are treatments for PPD using Chinese medicine. And of course, having a diagnosis helps with getting referrals to appropriate services and support, including getting insurance to cover your treatments.

Another condition that many of us new moms are prone to is post-traumatic stress disorder (PTSD). PTSD is usually linked to soldiers and survivors of abuse. Those are the stories that we hear most often. However, depending on how the pregnancy, labour, and birth experience went, any new mom can develop PTSD. Most important, any experience can be traumatic. One person's definition of traumatic will not be the same as the other.

It's worthwhile to talk to someone whenever you need to, even if you think it's a silly matter: your friends, family, support groups, health providers, counsellors, and therapists. There's usually a medical check-up for moms around week 6 postpartum where PPD screening is typically performed. This screening check may be done earlier and more frequently for new moms with a higher risk of PPD. I was also screened for PPD at each of my baby's wellness checks but that seemed more like a box to tick rather than a real check-in.

Overall, I feel that the current mental health screening efforts and preventive measures offered by modern medicine are grossly insufficient in ensuring a new mom's overall good health.

The modern health system needs to do more for new moms instead of just a one-time postpartum check-up for some countries or visits from midwives that are too short. It's inexcusable to let new moms just figure out when to ask for help. She's got enough to deal with in the Postpartum Year! But until policies change, this will remain the standard medical postpartum care for many.

"I view the avoidance of addressing emotions, fears, and doubts, during the first month when the hormonal, bodily, and life changes as detrimental to a mom's mental health and self-esteem."

—Dr. Pey Shyan, MBBS (Honours)

"I agree that emotions, fears and doubts should definitely be addressed and can definitely be harmful to a new mum's mental health and self-esteem. As we know, there is a growing movement around the world addressing women suffering birth trauma, some severe enough to have post-natal depression or psychotic episode. This should not be swept under the rug and should be addressed ASAP so as to ensure both physical and mental health of the new mother."

—Dr. Amanda Wee, MBBS, MRMed, MRANZCOG
Obstetrics and Gynaecology Advanced Trainee

What's reassuring for now is that there are emerging systems in local health communities that support new moms after leaving the hospital such as postpartum support groups lead by nurses and midwives. There are also doulas and therapists offering postpartum emotional support.

Recognising and addressing matrescence as a postpartum process is a good start. Providing specific support for new moms during matrescence would be the next step.

THE MODERN CONFINEMENT APPROACH FOR MANAGING EMOTIONS

My modern confinement philosophy for this part is as follows:

Your mind, soul, and heart
can only do so much alone
Ask for help when you need to
Accept help when it's offered to you
And most important,
EMBRACE YOUR EMOTIONS!

The first month after giving birth brings a wonderfully chaotic mess of emotions, including changes in hormones, the brutal exhaustion and sleep deprivation from tending to a newborn, and keeping up with the overnight transformation into a first-time mom, or a new mom of more children.

Having a good team to help you with your postpartum emotions can be a huge sanity saver. I highly suggest preparing for this before going into labour so that you can hash things out clearly with your support people before the wild postpartum hormones kick in hard.

Recall one of the TCM philosophies in the earlier section of this chapter about emotions and our health, *"Emotions become causes of disease when we do not 'possess them' but they 'possess us.'"*

I will never suggest suppressing your emotions. I'm an advocate for letting feelings wash over you. But after that, you're the one in control of the next step! Therefore, the recommendations I offer below is a version of "possessing" your emotions (i.e. you're ultimately the one in control of how you react and respond to your emotions).

For Moms

My recommendation for tackling emotions during the modern confinement month is to allow yourself to feel and seek a support person to unload your emotional baggage. I recommend doing this with another friend, a therapist, or your trusted support groups. This gives your confinement support person emotional space to perform their duties to you and watch over you.

If you do choose another friend to be your emotional baggage handler, do let this person know exactly what you're seeking from them:

- Do you want them to pity you just for that moment? *Hey, it's nice to hear someone echo that everything sucks for you right now even though you chose to have this child. It's just venting and releasing emotional tension. You're not a bad mother or an ungrateful person for feeling that way. You've got a lot going on right after birth and to make space for your true feelings to settle in, you've got to clear the confusion in the beginning.*
- Would you like them to offer solutions? Maybe you'd like positive reinforcements instead? What can they do if they feel overwhelmed by you?
- Being clear in what you expect from your friend prevents them from feeling overwhelmed.

If you have other ways you'd prefer to use to manage your heavy emotions, embrace them and get help to access them. These could be prayers—maybe you'd like to visit your church or temple once a week during confinement, listen to heavy metal, make healing visits to your trusted spiritualist, or spend time meditating with nature. Just remember to bundle up to keep warm and dry whenever you're out of the house!

CHECK-IN TIME!

DEAR NEW MOMS, YOU ARE NOT CRAZY! You are not a failure for allowing yourself to feel all the emotions. Actually, wait. I'll recant that. Yes, you are crazy for being so brave and embracing all those emotions! Crazy brave. It takes a lot of mental strength to acknowledge those emotions, hold them close, and carry them around with you until things settle down. I applaud you for being so courageous! Now, go and release them somewhere safe. And perform your closing ritual before you wind down. For example, you can do a simple deep breathing exercise while laying or sitting on the floor to ground yourself before heading back to your reality. Take a deep breath in as you imagine bright white light filling your lungs and spreading to the rest of your body. And as you exhale, imagine that white light turning brown and leaving your body through your feet or back. It's going straight into the ground, removing all the undesirable feelings and thoughts. Repeat 5 times and you're done!

For the Support Person

If you're a confinement support person, here's how you can support a new mom:

- Offer to be their emotional punching bag or emotional baggage handler. Your role is really to let them vent, complain, cry, yell, and not judge them for what they say and feel. Take it all from them and help them dump those emotions. They might have the darkest thoughts during this time but let them release those thoughts so that they may pass. Offer to create some kind of ritual or routine to close the session, if that works for both of you.

- Be tender. It's a volatile and vulnerable time for both of you. But remember, it's all about them just for this month. I promise that they're not an emotional wreck all the time. They need your help and love to wade through this month of huge, rapid changes.
- Listen, listen, and listen. To be clearer, you can ask them, "Would you like me to just listen, or do you want help finding solutions?"
- Be patient. They might go round in circles with the "same ol', same ol'" worries, but again, let them release those feelings as often as required so that those may pass.

SAFETY TIP

For new moms: Always reach out to your trusted friends and family and health professionals if you ever feel suicidal or have dark thoughts of harming yourself or your baby. You're not a bad person. You just need help.

For the confinement support person: Always check in on your loved one. Don't always accept their "I'm fine" answer because they may not want to admit they need help. New moms and moms in general tend to be bad at asking for help too. Notify health authorities if you're very worried about them having suicidal thoughts or thoughts of self-harm.

Have a list of emergency numbers for your local area and to your doctors or nurses clearly written and tacked to your fridge or somewhere easily accessible, and on speed-dial.

THE BARE NECESSITIES

- Rant. Vent. Complain. Laugh. Cry. Shout. Scream. Journal.
- I recommend choosing to feel and express your emotions whenever you're overwhelmed. This frees up some emotional space and energy for you to tackle the next day.

KEY THINGS TO REMEMBER

- Tackling the emotions that surface during this time can lead to a whole separate journey of self-discovery. It can be painful to some, liberating to others. Take this at your own pace.
- Help is always available. Have the courage to ask for it.
- Be selfish once in a while. We need to be nurtured so that we can be present and care for our babies.

INCLUDING YOUR PARTNER FROM PREGNANCY ONWARD

Now, let's explore how we can help modern dads, spouses, and partners be more included from pregnancy onward. Let's start normalising them playing important roles in births, the Postpartum Year, and in nurturing the young.

Historically, males and fathers weren't allowed into the birthing room and during confinement. Recall in the section "Chinese Cultural Views on Postpartum" in the introduction chapter. It was considered bad luck for fathers to come into contact with the birthing process. Meaning, bad luck will befall the family from then on if he did!

If we stick to this mindset today, I have no doubt that families will become more dysfunctional and postpartum depression will hit both moms and dads harder than ever. Why? The modern mom, who already shoulders so much mental and physical load caring for the newborn, will have to continue doing all the traditionally female-gendered tasks while trying to thrive in a modern world. The resentment and feelings of guilt and failure will undoubtedly permeate both parties.

The ongoing exclusion of fathers, spouses, and partners can also increase the risk of them developing postpartum depression. Yes! Fathers and males CAN get postpartum depression too.

POSTPARTUM PATERNAL DEPRESSION

Postpartum paternal depression can happen anytime within the Postpartum Year (anytime within the first year of having a baby).

How does this happen? If a new mom has postpartum depression or a history of depressive disorders, then their spouses and partners are at risk for depression too. It's really not easy to help someone through depression. And it can hurt more knowing that their wife and mother of their children is hurting but they can't easily fix things for her. This can also be a reminder of how "useless" spouses and partners perceive themselves to be during pregnancy, labour, and birth. And unfortunately, the majority of fathers may not have many strong social support systems for them to express their emotions and worries.

There's also the anxiety about becoming a first-time dad. Or having more children. The stress of wanting to be a good and better father, husband, and partner. And a lot of that anxiety likely stems from them trying to break away from the patriarchal norms that still permeate our modern society. Our modern men and fathers are also cycle breakers of their generation as much as the modern women and moms are for theirs.

Therefore, in my modern confinement practice, fathers, spouses, and partners are encouraged to be the main confinement support person in place of moms and MILs. Let's learn how to include them in your modern confinement practice.

Regardless of whether you'd like to do a traditional confinement or follow my modern version, here are practical ways to include fathers, spouses, and partners in your postpartum practice. Naturally, this works best when both of you design the postpartum plan together!

Here are some areas where fathers, spouses, and partners can play a big role in the confinement month and for the rest of the Postpartum Year:

- Food preparation or meal preparation so that the entire family has meals ready to go for the week.
- Serving the new mother during the confinement month: Bring her meals, teas, and soups!
- Baby care: Especially at night, it's mighty helpful to get the baby ready for mom to nurse or feed the baby. During those 6 to 8 weeks when the new mom is in recovery, it's painful and uncomfortable enough for her to waddle and hobble from the bed to the bathroom in the middle of the night. So give her a sense of security by changing the baby's diaper or soothing the baby until she's ready for the baby.
- Cleaning, errands, and caring for the other children: The new mom should really only be carrying the

newborn during her recovery. Anything heavier than the baby or tasks requiring exertion of the abdominal core should be performed by someone else! Yes, that includes vacuuming, mopping, caring for the other children, and doing the dishes; because standing for long periods of time requires activation of the core muscles. So does chasing after the other children, especially if they're toddlers. And the new mom should really be resting rather than doing dishes and caring for the other children! Here's where fathers, spouses, and partners can really make a difference to a new mom's recovery and also for the dynamics of the family. Taking over these tasks might seem trivial but it's really keeping the entire household together and running smoothly. And the other children will learn by example that mom needs rest and how to help her get the rest she needs!

At the end of the day, both of you will find ways to include fathers, spouses, and partners as you walk through planning your modern confinement month. Because every family's needs are unique.

With that said, let's start planning your modern confinement month tailored to your needs!

Chapter 9

Personalising Your Confinement Practice

Why is it important to personalise your modern confinement practice?

Your needs, circumstances, and limitations are unique to you. While generalised plans can help you, it's unlikely that you'll reap the most benefit. This is why social media accounts and businesses that appeal to specific groups of people or situations have such a strong following, because they're able to offer advice and recommendations that are specific to unique challenges.

Personalising your confinement practice means you're able to include, exclude, and adjust things to help you achieve the postpartum recovery and experience that you want. But first, let's understand the definition of health. You'd be surprised how each of us views it differently.

WHAT IS HEALTH?

In this book, I've been following the World Health Organization (WHO) definition of health: *"Health is a state of complete physical, mental and social well-being and not merely the absence of disease or infirmity."*

It's very important to understand this definition because many of us have been brought up to view good health mainly as the absence of an illness. Or that having good physical health is sufficient. In reality, to be in a state of good health, we must be fulfilled in all aspects described in the quote above plus not be ill. Now, let's apply this definition to ourselves as new moms.

Once we've given birth and physically recovered, and assuming we don't have any other health conditions, we're technically healthy, right? Since we don't have any illness. But what about the anxiety we feel as a first-time mom or a new mom to more children? The insecurity we feel in our postpartum body? The worry about how to step out of the home for simple chores with a newborn? The loneliness of motherhood that many of us tend to feel from time to time or all the time for some? The pressure of being the Super Mom and juggling childcare, housekeeping, self-care, and work (for working moms)?

So, do we usually have good health in the Postpartum Year? Following WHO's definition, no, most of us don't! Our mental and social well-being aren't well looked after although physically we might have recovered. Although gender roles are shifting and the modern dad is more active in childcare and chores, moms still carry the bulk of housekeeping, looking after the family, and the mental load of keeping everything and everyone in check on top of their own workload and ambitions.

Will we ever have good health?

The hope is, yes! But that'll likely take much longer to achieve on a larger scale since we've got to rely on governments, policies, and other authorities and organisations to step in and pull their weight to make better care for moms the new standard. For now, we can take this small step and personalise a postpartum recovery month. Most important, we're able to do this by ourselves and with the help of our loved ones and community.

Now that we understand our health includes the physical, mental, emotional, and having a good social support system, let's look at a guide map to help you personalise your modern confinement practice.

You can flex your creativity here and design an experience that fits you. There's also space to include your confinement support person and other loved ones if you wish to.

GUIDE MAP TO PERSONALISING YOUR MODERN CONFINEMENT PRACTICE

1. Set ONE Main Confinement Goal and Manage Expectations

It's helpful to do the related exercise so that you'll have a guide for the next few steps in personalising your confinement practice. The best way is to KISS! Keep It Super Simple! As much as possible, of course. So, if you haven't already done it, hop back to chapter 3 and complete the exercise.

2. Decide on a Confinement Style: Traditional, Modern, or the Bare Necessities

This is not a reflection of your lifestyle. Your confinement style is how you'd like to follow the confinement practice. Do you want to go full-traditional? Or would you like to have a modern version (which I've defined in the beginning as a confinement practice that works with your modern lifestyle and needs while following certain confinement rules). This is completely your choice. Deciding on this part is separate from your main confinement goal and expectations.

Traditional Confinement

This style will follow the stricter ways of confinement. 30 days. No baths, showers, or washing hair during this period. In terms of entertainment, I recommend no social media, no TV, and no reading, but listening to music, podcasts, and audiobooks related to feel-good content is allowed. Journaling is also a good idea for emotional moments. However, I do not recommend following the traditional confinement principle of suppressing emotions. I encourage you to embrace, explore, and talk about them if and when you need to. Refer to chapter 8 for details. Food and beverage-wise, be strict with eating and drinking only warm food and beverages as per the advice of your TCM provider. It's always worth asking a TCM provider what foods (that are accessible in your area) are warm in nature. Always keep warm but not to the extent of sweating. Avoid all air-conditioning and direct drafts from fans and open windows. Wear long-sleeved clothes if you have to go out. Preferably, stay home for all 30 days.

Modern Confinement

This style involves adjusting certain traditional confinement rules to be easier to follow in our modern lifestyle. We're still sticking to the 30 days. This time frame also works with our modern work calendars and leave time.

- With showers and hair washing, that depends on how modernised you'd like to be. You can choose the fully modern approach where you can shower and wash your hair right after giving birth. Otherwise, you can compromise. Follow the traditional style for 2 weeks then modern for the rest of your confinement month. See chapter 6 for more on this.

- With food and beverages, stick to warm foods and drinks. If you crave cold stuff, have them at room temperature rather than iced. Personally, I have cheat days. I allow myself one small cup of something iced or cooled in the fridge when I really want to satisfy a craving for something chilled. On really hot days, this can be tricky. The best compromise is to still have room temperature beverages. I recommend chatting with your TCM provider about how to mitigate this. While you may consciously choose to have cold foods and drinks, and are sure that you won't worry about doing that, your subconscious might think otherwise. This can cause you to fret and feel guilty for giving in to cravings.

The Bare Necessities

This confinement version is for the busiest of us and for those of us with the least amount of support to be able to carry out the full confinement experience. I recommend focusing on the following to gain some benefit of the confinement practice by following the bare necessities from each section:

Warmth: Keep warm for 30 days. This means wearing long-sleeved clothes and keeping your neck warm with a scarf, especially during cold seasons and if your work place usually runs cold or is exposed to draughty, windy weather. If it's really warm, sweating is inevitable so hydrate, hydrate, hydrate! For both cold and hot environments, keep away from sitting under air conditioners and away from fans blowing directly at you.

No ice cream and cold drinks and food! Anything warm and room temperature is fine to consume. But as above in the modern confinement section, it can get tricky to avoid cold drinks and food on really hot days. I recommend chatting with your TCM provider about how to mitigate this.

Wind: Focus on avoiding Wind buildup in the body and expelling Wind that's already in the body. Ginger in foods and teas. Ginger is great for expelling gas from your body. Brewing teas with ginger and boiling soups with ginger is an easy way to keep ginger in your diet for 30 days.

Avoid "windy" foods. These are foods that cause gas to build up in your body. Beans, lentils, broccoli, cabbage, milk, and cheese are among those foods that make you fart a lot.

Rest: This is going to be tough for those of you who have a lot going on and don't have much help. Or if you have to go back to work early. But whenever you can, rest. This part will take a lot of creativity to sneak in rest and sleep time, so I highly recommend brainstorming with your bosses, managers, friends, and loved ones to figure out how to carve out time for you to rest. Here are some ideas, but you'll have to see if it really works for you. And if you can, adjust the ideas to your needs and situation.

Freeze your meals as much in advance as you can. Or buy frozen meals. Then all you need to do is stick them in the oven or microwave.

Catch up on sleep and rest on the weekends and days off. Engage your network for this. Have you got friends and family who can help with chores and look after the kids? Maybe a nonprofit around your area offers respite childcare for new moms who have to go back to work early? Even a 2-hour nap is better than nothing. But it can get tricky to get rest and sleep!

Turn chores into organised mess. Maybe you don't need to fold your laundry. Maybe you can just label the laundry baskets as JEANS, T-SHIRTS, UNDIES, and so on, and just chuck those cleaned clothes into those baskets. Maybe your kitchen always seems to be a mess. That's okay. Let the dishes pile up. You can block out a day of the week to tackle the kitchen if that works. If not, try to wash things as you finish with them if you're not too tired!

Emotions: Feel. Embrace them. Vent. Release. Take a deep breath. And perform your closing ritual. Get a blank journal specific for your postpartum recovery time and pour anything and everything you want into it. If you've got friends and family, or a therapist or counsellor, who are able to help you decompress emotionally, please engage them for help. This is crucial to your mental and emotional health.

3. Check Logistics

In this part of your confinement planning, we'll look at four main areas that can affect how you'll carry out your confinement practice.

Finances

For those who don't have paid parental leave, can you afford to take 30 days off? Can your spouse or partner afford to take 30 days off with you? Can you afford buying special Chinese ingredients and herbs in bulk? Or do you have to do a weekly shop instead? Can you afford to hire a doula or nighttime nanny when you need extra help? Can you afford the occasional cleaning person to help clean your home during the 30 days or Fourth Trimester? Is it cost-effective to subscribe to a food delivery service like HelloFresh?

Ingredients Access

Are there Chinese or Asian shops close to you that sell herbs and spices? Or can you only access them online? Do they deliver? Do they even have the herbs that you need? Do the local grocery stores have the ingredients you need for cooking confinement foods?

TCM Access

Are there TCM clinics in your area? Do they also stock herbs at their clinic? If there's none within driving distance around you, are there clinics you can visit in another state? Or call to get a phone consultation? Can you order herbs from them to deliver to your home? Or are there TCM practitioners that have embraced telehealth and offer online consultations?

4. Complete Home Review

I recommend reviewing the previous chapters that were divided into areas of your home when preparing for your confinement practice: the kitchen, bathroom, living room, bedroom, and the outdoors. Reviewing your main confinement goal while walking through these areas can help you see better how to make things functional for your recovery month. For example, if your main confinement goal is "to have peace," then you could prepare the following areas in your home to meet that goal:

Kitchen

Allow dishes to stack up. One day a week is focused on cleaning the kitchen and all the dishes. Allocate a person to do this task and it shouldn't be the new mom. Try to wash dishes and utensils as they're being used. But the priority is to have an organised mess and not argue over the dishes.

Bathroom

Make sure all hygiene products the new mom needs are in stock. This means she has everything she needs within reach, reducing the chance of her feeling frustrated that something is out when she's finished or just started using the toilet.

Bedroom

Organised mess! With the main goal of peace, that means less clutter too. But knowing how difficult it is to keep cleaning all the time, we can still keep the clutter at bay by organising the mess. Make piles along the sides of the room if that's what works for you. Most important, the bed where the new mom is resting on is comfortable, clean, and free of clutter. And make sure there's tissues or clean face towels, water, snacks, and phone charger on her bedside table.

Living Room

Organised mess once more to maintain the peace and keep clutter at bay! If you've got other children (and pets), this can be a tough one. There are two main things in this area that can be done to achieve the confinement goal of peace:

- Once the new mom has chosen her area for rest and nursing in the living room, keep this couch/chair/ area clean and comfortable. Pillows, blanket, towels, snacks, water, and phone charger at the minimum so that this area is functional for the new mom to rest.
- The rest of the living room? Just have boxes to pile things into so that it makes clean-up quick and easy. Having some clear space can do wonders for everyone's mental health.

Baby Supplies

Have a portable box or bag with all the baby necessities—diapers, wipes, baby powder/barrier cream, some clothes, burp cloths, and pacifier if you're using one. Why have a bag or box of these supplies when you're at home? So that you don't have to go searching for it when you need to change your baby! You can carry this bag or box around the house and know that everything you need is in there. You can also place a box of baby supplies in each main room. But from my experience, the chaos in my home means that these supplies don't stay in the same spot! I find having them "follow me" around the house was a lot more useful and less stressful than needing to constantly find stuff.

Guide Table for Personalising Your Confinement Practice

Step 1: Overarching Review of My Confinement Practice	My Love Language:
	My Main Confinement Goal:
	My Top 3 Expectations for My Confinement Month:
	What's the weather like during my confinement month? Summer or Spring/Hot or Winter or Fall/Cold

Step 2: Logistics Review	Finances	• Can we afford to have a full 30-day confinement month? • Can my spouse/partner take 30 days time off from work to care for me? Or a partial confinement experience? • Can we afford to hire a doula or confinement nanny for 30 days straight? Or for a few days during the 30 days?
	Ingredients Access	• Can we find the Chinese herbal ingredients locally for my confinement teas and soups? Or do we have to order online or make a special trip to buy them? • Can we find the Asian ingredients locally to cook the types of confinement foods I want? Or do we have to order online or make a special trip to buy them?
	TCM Access	• Can we find a TCM doctor and herbalist close to home? • Or do we have to make do with a phone or online consultation? • Or make a special trip to the nearest available TCM specialist before our baby arrives?

Step 3: My Confinement Style	Based on the above reviews, My Chosen Style for Confinement is TRADITIONAL or MODERN

Step 4: Home Review Based on My Confinement Style	Kitchen	How do I set things up FUNCTIONALLY in these areas to meet my recovery and daily needs?
	Bathroom	• Setting things up functionally means arranging things in that area so that it's easy for you, the one recovering from giving birth, to get things done for yourself and your newborn.
	Bedroom	• For breastfeeding moms, this can look like having a small bucket of snacks with a bottle of water in all the areas you would nurse your baby.
	Living Room	• Or having all your socks in a bucket by the front door so that you don't end up running back and forth to your bedroom if you forget your socks!
	Outdoors	

MANAGING SETBACKS DURING YOUR CONFINEMENT

Setbacks can feel like you don't want to continue with the confinement practice anymore during the 30 days. Setbacks can also happen before you start your confinement, such as having an unplanned C-section or any other health conditions that occur due to the unpredictable nature of labour and birth.

First, if you're unable to start your confinement practice the day after you've given birth for any reason, I recommend starting whenever you can. This takes away the stress of being strict with the timeline of a traditional confinement. Additionally, depending on the country you're living in, some hospitals prefer to discharge you and your newborn 2 to 3 days after you've given birth. You can start following the nutrition aspect of your confinement practice plan while in hospital but if that's inconvenient, then just start when you get home!

Next, we'll address how to stay the course with your confinement practice and prevent frustration and poor motivation to continue:

Stay Consistent

Make a list of daily confinement tasks you've chosen to follow. Tick them off as you complete them. Allow yourself space to complete the tasks however is easiest for you. You could have a routine you follow. Or you could perform the tasks anytime during the day that works for you depending on your responsibilities of the day. You could also combine both methods! No matter how you choose to carry out the confinement tasks, as long as you stick to completing them each day, that counts as being consistent. And being consistent can build "muscle memory" so if you happen to miss a task, you might feel "off" until you complete it.

Celebrate Small Wins Every Day

Maybe reward yourself with a confinement friendly snack after ticking off all your confinement tasks for the day. Identifying daily small wins that help can be easier to do when you've identified your love languages. This will definitely help you fill your emotional bucket and, therefore, give you the motivation to stick to it till the end of the 30 days!

Reward Yourself for Completing Your Confinement Month

Oh, this was my favourite way to help me power through all the confinement foods and drinks! I visualised sitting at my favourite buffet place, eating everything and anything I wanted after I was done with my confinement. You could reward yourself with anything that suits your fancy. It doesn't have to be about food! Maybe a shopping spree of some sort. Maybe donate to your favourite charity.

Plan a Party after Confinement

(See chapter 10 about celebrations after confinement.) Planning for a party, big or small, can help distract you from that itchy scalp or feeling warm. Walk around your home to see what the party would look like. What will the baby wear? What will you wear? What kind of food and drinks would you like to serve? Will you be cooking or ordering for the party? Oh, so much to scheme and plan for!

Schedule Cheat Days

Allow one day a week for a small cheat window. Have some cheat foods and drinks that you'll be comfortable consuming without feeling a ton of guilt. Take this cheat day if you need it and then go back to your routine and plan. At least you've got this to tide you over if you really feel like you need to break out of your confinement plan once in a while.

If you're feeling really frustrated, burned out, and poorly motivated during your confinement month despite trying the above, stop. Breathe. Have a full day of doing whatever you need and want. And reset the next day. Debrief with your support person and review the confinement plan if needed. Call your TCM provider if they've been involved with your confinement planning and ask for advice on tweaking things or how to keep pushing forward.

NOTE TO SPOUSES, PARTNERS, FRIENDS, AND FAMILY MEMBERS

Whether you're the designated confinement support person or not, helping your loved one stick to their confinement plan is very much needed. If you're feeling extra supportive, follow the confinement month rituals and tasks with the new mom from day one! This is going to help so much because you're able to empathise with your loved one's discomfort and you can complain together.

My husband ate whatever I ate and didn't snack on things I wasn't allowed to. I appreciate him so much for that. He also avoided watching emotional and horror shows during that time. The downside was he picked a comedy show during my second confinement while I was in a lot of pain from my C-section wound. Laughing so much hurt me so bad, I cried. We laugh about it now (painlessly!) every time we think back to that moment.

PREPARING FOR MEDICAL COMPLICATIONS

Imagine after all that planning and gah! You have to have an emergency C-section, you've got a high risk of developing blood clots post-surgery, and your blood pressure remains high hours later and even once you're back home. Or worse, you develop some difficult complication that requires intensive care and days in the hospital.

Confinement during Recovery

Can you still practice a confinement month if you've got a lot to recover from? Yes, you can! I'd recommend working closely with both your modern health practitioner and your TCM practitioner to ensure your recovery isn't conflicted by assumptions such as the following:

"I think these herbs are still fine to take although I've had a lot of bleeding at the hospital."

"Oh man, I think I better just throw my confinement plan out the window since I didn't have a vaginal birth."

Adjusting Your Confinement Practice Plan for an Emergency

The priority is to recover your health if you're having or had a medical and/or surgical emergency related to your pregnancy and birth (or if you suddenly develop a health complication during the 6 to 8 weeks after giving birth).

Your recovery is the most important thing because without you being in decent health, you won't be able to practice much of a confinement month let alone care for your newborn. And by decent health, I mean the bare minimum of good health. Meaning you're able to eat and drink, your bowels are moving (you're not constipated) and you're well hydrated, and you're not in danger of tipping into another medical emergency while recovering at home.

While your physical health takes precedence at this stage, having a bare necessities confinement plan still allows you to exert some control over your recovery. And it reminds your loved ones that you're still a priority just like your newborn is. Finally, for those of you who worry about not completing a confinement practice in full due to your health, a bare necessities confinement will allow you to fulfill this tradition and receive benefits.

So, I highly recommend following the bare necessities confinement style in this case. Here are two general situations you may come across and my recommendations on planning for them.

1. You have a smooth pregnancy and don't expect complications during birth.

In this case, I recommend having a backup confinement plan following the bare minimum style in case you have an emergency C-section.

MY STORY

I didn't have a backup confinement plan to match my needs for recovery after a C-section. I managed to adjust my plan but it took me about a week to clarify certain information and it added stress I didn't need. When in doubt, ring your TCM health provider and ask them about any uncertainties you have. What I did was ask my OBGYN team about any herbal contraindications for C-sections (stuff I couldn't take), what foods and drinks I was limited to while recovering, and what health risks I needed to be careful about because of having a major surgery (for example, sudden bleeding, infection at my wound, and risk of developing clots in my legs). Then, I brought this information to my TCM pharmacist to get her advice on how to adjust the herbs I took.

---

2. You're expecting a challenging birth and/or are having a planned C-section.

If this is you, I recommend focusing on creating your bare minimum confinement plan first. Then design your ideal confinement practice. This way, you know you have a confinement practice that works to your unique yet challenging situation. And if things go smoother than expected, you get to add on the confinement practices from your ideal plan! Make sure to also engage your modern and TCM health provider early on when planning for this.

Planning a Backup Confinement Practice

1. Are the herbs you're using safe for consumption after a major surgery? Ask your TCM doctor or TCM pharmacist.

2. Focus on dispelling wind and gas. Modern health providers are likely to prescribe you medication to remove gas buildup in your abdomen after a C-section. Add on ginger drinks and food to help that along.

3. Focus on rest with some light moving about. Yes, you have to rest but you've also got to keep mobile! Take short walks around the house. Keeping mobile can prevent constipation and maintain some muscle mass in your body. It's also really important to move about to avoid clots from forming in your leg veins.

4. Hydrate, hydrate, hydrate. After giving birth, having a major surgery, or having a major medical intervention, your body really needs a lot of rehydration while recovering at home. Healing wounds take a lot out of our bodies so we need to hydrate to maintain the healing process. And making sure you're able to poo without straining much is very important for recovery in general!

5. Ask, ask, ask. Engage your modern and TCM health providers early on! This is also a good opportunity to get more education on what to expect after giving birth. Besides doctors and nurse practitioners, the

OBGYN nurses, midwives, and doulas are also great resources on learning more about the postpartum recovery time and the rest of the Postpartum Year.

Why You Should Prepare for the Worst

Why am I addressing this can of worms? Why are we planning for an emergency? Don't you have enough to worry about? Let's face it. Not talking about your worries only makes them worse, especially with your pregnancy, birth, and life after that. I know because I've tried ignoring my worries and "just focusing on the positive!" (very much like how Joy from the Pixar film *Inside Out* kept trying to suppress and ignore Sadness only for things to go from bad to worse) during my first pregnancy and, well, that just made my anxiety worse.

Once I started talking to my OBGYN and the birthing suite nurses about my concerns and curiosities, a huge weight lifted off my shoulders. I even asked my OBGYN what their protocol was for postpartum haemorrhage (PPH) because all the pregnancy and birth-related complications I learned about in medical school and saw during my OBGYN term came flooding back to me. I'm glad I asked him because he understood where my anxiety was coming from (knowing and having seen too much as a doctor!) and he happily gave me a rundown of how they handled PPH at their hospital.

HOW TO RAISE YOUR CONCERNS
WITH YOUR HEALTHCARE PROVIDER

Having been on both sides of the hospital bed (as a doctor and as a patient), I'd recommend the following whenever you have even the slightest concern about your pregnancy, birth, and/or postpartum health:

- Always MAKE A LIST. The pregnancy brain fog is real. The postpartum "mom brain" is also real. Why? Your body is way too busy growing a baby and then recovering from 9 months of that plus healing from giving birth. It's no surprise that the majority of your energy is diverted away from less important functions such as thinking and remembering things.

- Always go through your list with your health provider at every visit. Bring a pen to write down answers.

- Ask for a list of resources if your health provider has recommendations that they think might help you. Ask them to email you, print it for you, or write down the details for you.

- If you don't understand the information in any resource given to you, ask someone from your health provider's team to clarify your questions. You can also speak to your general practitioner or family medicine specialist if you have access to them. Nurse practitioners are also a good source of knowledge.

- If you don't feel like your worries have been addressed adequately, reframe the question. Sometimes, your health provider hasn't switched mental gears from clinical to layperson. If you still don't feel satisfied, talk to another health provider in the same team. This can be the nurse, ultrasonographer, and allied health members like physiotherapists and nutritionists. You can also speak to a social worker or patient liaison officer (or similar) to escalate your concerns if that's necessary.

For my second pregnancy, I wasn't as worried about the birth since I'd "been there, done that." I also did well without an epidural with my first because I'm afraid of it (yes, I'm more afraid of the epidural than the contraction pains). So, I completely brushed off the idea that I should talk about my fear of emergency C-sections and epidurals with my OBGYN this time around. That meant that I did not prepare myself emotionally and mentally for the probability of those events occurring and I didn't allocate space in my confinement plan for a C-section recovery.

But as Murphy's Law states, "Anything that can go wrong will go wrong." So, of course my second birth went pear-shaped with me ending up needing an emergency C-section. It was a nightmare come true for me that day. I suppose the signs were there in the beginning because the German hospital I was supposed to go to didn't have midwives available the night we showed up. I was walking up and down the hospital corridors at around 1:00 a.m. with a toddler in tow because my husband was walking ahead trying to get things organised for me. They had to transfer me to another hospital while I was already 5 cm dilated.

A PERSONAL STORY:
MY EMERGENCY C-SECTION
WAS A NIGHTMARE COME TRUE

As a final year medical student in University of Queensland, Australia, I had to do an OBGYN term. During my first couple of weeks at the regional hospital I was posted to, I was told by the OBGYN surgeon, "I need you to be my first-assist in our patient's emergency C-section. We don't have enough residents today." This was the first patient I was assigned to learn how to deliver babies. We had to "catch" 5 babies at the very least by the end of our term.

I always had a fear of pregnancy and birth, so I didn't read about how C-sections happened in detail. I knew the gist of it from pre-clinical studies. I mean, what were the chances of me being directly involved as a student? I was one of those medical students who knew early on that I had zero interest in any specialty that was surgically related. And I made that clear to my instructors. I figured I'd just observe a C-section at the most.

Well, it happened anyway! First-assist to the OBGYN surgeon meant I was directly opposite her, pulling and pushing, grunting and huffing, during the super quick procedure given it was an emergency C-section. Was this dangerous to the patient? No, because the doctor I was with was a very experienced surgeon and she needed me mainly for the additional manpower for certain things.

She did all the incisions and stitching; navigating the organs, nerves, and blood vessels; and retrieving the placenta. The baby's face popped out as soon as the surgeon opened our patient's uterus and then we applied pressure to the top of her belly to push the baby out.

But gosh! I can say I was pretty traumatised after that. C-sections are ROUGH. I thought, "I'll NEVER willingly choose a C-section, so I better not have kids!"

So, being awake for my emergency C-section meant that everything I saw on the other side of the sheet as the OBGYN surgeon's first-assist many years ago came flooding back to me.

I could clearly visualise every incision pressure, tug and pull, and the feeling of my baby coming out of my uterus as though I was helping operate on myself. To say I was terrified is an understatement. I cried so hard when I realised I had to have an emergency C-section and the medical team thought it was because I felt bad I couldn't have a vaginal birth.

But no. I cried because I had to live a nightmare. I totally blindsided myself by not preparing myself mentally beforehand for the possibility of a C-section! And I couldn't choose not to do it because my baby had started showing distress on the foetal monitor. That was a clear indication to get my baby out as soon as possible for her life and safety.

I tell you this story to empower and encourage you to acknowledge your worries and fears, and to talk about them. I give you permission to be afraid. And to ask as many questions as you want! Your pregnancy and birth stories will stick with you for life—mentally, emotionally, and physically. And to recap, we also know that pregnancies and births have a mind of their own! You can try as hard as possible to have the smoothest pregnancy and best birth experience. But the reality is, things will happen the way they want to.

So, you have every right to worry and be scared if you need to be. Acknowledging these worries and fears will allow you to find some answers that can lift you and prepare you emotionally and mentally for the birth.

I'll take this further to say that considering emergencies and planning a backup confinement practice can help alleviate some of this anxiety and fear because you're taking back some control amidst all the chaos. This can also help you through your recovery and postpartum journey because you are less likely to be blindsided by your emotions and expectations if the unexpected happens.

Then, at the end of the messy birthing and recovery tunnel, there's the bright light of parties and celebrations waiting for you and baby!

Chapter 10

Celebrations after Confinement

There are two celebrations my mom held for my babies after my confinement month: the full-moon celebration (30 days after birth or after the confinement period) and the 100th day celebration.

Many families today tend to favour the 100th day celebration, throwing grand parties and feasts; some even host a banquet at a hotel ballroom! They'll usually practice traditions that are performed with the full-moon event during this time. There are also party event planners in Malaysia, Singapore, and Hong Kong that offer the 100th day celebration package and services. It's that popular!

But overall, it depends on what your family tradition is.

Let's learn more about these celebrations!

THE FULL MOON CELEBRATION

Traditionally, the Chinese consider the full 30 days after birth as the first birthday of a newborn or baby's "full-moon" known as *man yue* (满月). This is equivalent to a full lunar cycle from new moon to full moon—about 30 days. This also marks the end of the new mom's confinement period and she's now able to bathe and wash her hair and emerge from her room.

Naturally, this calls for a celebration! It's also the perfect time for families to present their baby to the public because both mom and baby have passed the vulnerable period.

BABY'S 100TH DAY CELEBRATION

This tradition stems from the imperial ancient Chinese days as described in the *Book of Rites* section on "The Pattern of the Family."[27] As mentioned earlier in this book, the *Book of Rites* or *Liji* is an ancient text that informs the elite aristocrats of ancient China about Confucian rituals and practices.

At the end of the infant's third month of life, equivalent to about 100 days, the baby's hair is shaved off in gender-specific styles: a pair of horn-like tufts of hair are left behind for boys, and a circular tuft of hair is left behind on the crown for girls. There is another hair style used where a portion of hair is left on the left of the boy's head, and on the right for the girls. Shaving of a baby's hair is believed to remove the "polluted foetal hair,"[28] which is considered unlucky.

27. "Full Moon: Celebrating One of Baby's First Milestones," Singapore Motherhood, last modified 12 July, 2016, https://singaporemotherhood.com/full-moon-man-yue-baby-celebration-singapore-tradition.
28. "The Book of Rites, The Birth of a Child," World History Commons, https://worldhistorycommons.org/book-rites-birth-child.

Then, after mom and baby cleanse themselves with a bath, both are presented to the father and later, to the rest of the family. Essentially, these rites were performed to mark the infant's developing relationship with the father and entrance into society.

TRADITIONAL CELEBRATION PRACTICES[29]

Bathing for Mom and Baby

Traditionally, the confinement month meant no bathing and washing hair for mom and baby following birth. So, once the confinement was over, mom and baby would have a cleansing ritual to wash off all the unlucky "pollution" of childbirth before meeting the father and rest of the family. But in our modern times, this tradition has evolved to something optional for mom and baby to do if that's their wish or family tradition. In Malaysia, some Chinese families will soak pomelo leaves in the bath water for mom and baby to use for washing. Pomelo leaves in Chinese culture are believed to have cleansing powers and can ward off evil and bad luck. My mother used to prepare bath water with pomelo leaves for us to wash in on Chinese New Year Eve for this very reason.

Red Clothes and Gold Jewellery

This practice is part of the presentation of the newborn and mom to the family's ancestors and the deities they worship. For those who don't perform such rituals, wearing red and adorning a baby in gold accessories is still part of blessing the child with good luck, prosperity, and success.

---

29. "The Book of Rites, The Birth of a Child."

Red-Dyed Hard-Boiled Eggs

Hard-boiled eggs signify new birth and renewal of life (including new beginnings!) and are dyed red for good luck. These are gifted to family members and friends to share in the good vibes!

Pickled Ginger

This condiment tastes sour. In the Cantonese language, the word "sour" sounds like "grandson." Since boys tended to be preferred over girls back in the day (and still are to some degree today), this condiment is served alongside the hard-boiled eggs to hope for more grandsons. Unfortunately, there's no equivalent dish for girls.

> I personally view this as sexist and did not have this condiment at my girls' celebrations. It brings a sour note (pun intended) to a joyous event. Why should I be thinking of having and wishing for sons when I've just started celebrating and enjoying my baby girl? But if you'd like to include this or find a substitute with a less sexist meaning, have a chat to your elders and ask for advice.

Baby's First Haircut

Some families still shave off baby's hair at their full-moon or on the 100th day celebration. The modern belief is that a baby's hair will grow back thicker and stronger. Some families just snip off a lock of hair, tie it with red string, and store it as a keepsake.

CELEBRATIONS FOR THE MODERN FAMILY

Nowadays (in the twenty-first century), many families choose to celebrate either the full-moon or the 100th day. Some choose to celebrate both. It's entirely up to you and your family! It's also up to you how grand you'd like to have it.

For my little family, we held a very intimate full-moon celebration. For my first child, my mother and brother stayed with my husband and me for my confinement month, so it was just 5 of us (including baby!). For my second child, only my husband and I and our eldest celebrated baby number 2's full-moon. For my baby's 100th day, we had extended family and friends over for a larger party with more food. We also dressed up the baby in red clothes and adorned her with gold jewellery gifted by my Malaysian family members.

If you'd like to host your baby's 100th day celebration after a full-moon event, I would recommend having a smaller, intimate full-moon party with immediate family members and then a larger 100th day celebration. This way, the party preparations and cost will be manageable, and it won't be too crowded around your baby (unless you have a large immediate family!). Your immediate family can also carry out the new-born and end-of-confinement rituals in peace without all the chaos of a large party.

Another modern twist is to celebrate mom as much as the baby during these events. Maybe have her go to a spa (if she's recovered well enough for that) or for a light massage before the celebration. Gift her a hair salon visit, complete with scalp and shoulder massage during a wonderful hair wash and hair treatment session. Goodness knows my visits to the hair salon after my confinement for a session like the above made me feel so DARNED GOOD! Mainly because I spent 2 weeks not washing my hair and having a good scrub was heavenly. I also went for a facial, manicure, and pedicure just because I felt like it. Then, when we had those post-confinement celebrations, oh I felt so wonderful, pampered, mostly healed, and happy! Most important, celebrate mom the way she'd like. Remember, the postpartum recovery month is all about mom, so celebrating the end of that is also about her.

So remember, adjusting traditional celebrations to what our modern family needs and wants doesn't mean we're disrespecting our ancestors and heritage. As long as we're doing it thoughtfully and making these changes together with our elders, we're able to keep tradition alive for the future generation.

Celebration Ideas

I recommend having red-dyed hard-boiled eggs at the very least regardless of how you'd like to celebrate this event. Even if you're not throwing a party, having these red-dyed eggs just for you and your partner and/or kids marks the end of confinement and baby's full moon. Since hard-boiled eggs signify new birth and renewal of life (including new beginnings!) and are dyed red for good luck, it's the best and simplest dish to have at the end of your confinement month.

A CHILDHOOD MEMORY

My mother always made sure we ate hard-boiled eggs with the shell dyed red every year on our birthdays (following the Chinese lunar calendar). Even after I've moved overseas and lived by myself, she'd always text me the day before my Chinese lunar birthdate and remind me to make these for myself. And specifically 2 eggs! Why? Double the good luck for new beginnings as I started another year of life!

Sticking to the spirit of this book on modernising traditions thoughtfully with our elders, here are some party recommendations if the traditional methods aren't convenient or relevant to your access to resources and ingredients. My mom helped a lot with party ideas in this section. These are also fun for families with mixed Asian-Western cultures. You get to combine both!

Baby Shower-Inspired Celebration

The United States loves throwing baby showers for parents-to-be before the baby is born. It's a trend that's growing in many places but it's not a common Asian tradition. But if you'd like to have an America- or Western-themed celebration, you can choose to celebrate the full-moon or 100th day like a baby shower.

This means finger food, gifts for mom and baby, and games! My husband's side is American, and my sister-in-law organised a baby shower for us. Naturally, my recommendations below are American in nature.

Menu suggestions: cupcakes, cookies, fries, sausages or hot dogs, sodas, fruit punch, cheese platters, raw veggies with dip, crackers with dip, nachos, chips and dip

Games suggestions:

- Guess the Flavour in the Diaper: Smear baby food flavours and/or popular favourites like peanut butter and Nutella onto diapers. Have guests put their guesses onto a card and whoever has the most correct answers wins! It's up to guests how they'd like to decipher the flavours. This ends up being very hilarious to watch!
- Pregnant Belly Challenge: Attach balloons to the front of guests' stomachs and have them compete over who can tie their shoelaces the fastest. It's a close experience to trying to put on shoes with a very pregnant belly!

Hotpot Meal

Malaysians (well, most East Asians) love our steamboat or hotpot meals. It's really nice to have everyone sit around the hotpot to cook and eat together. It's also easy to prepare and clean up. So, to make things easy for an intimate meal, you can throw a hotpot party!

Menu Suggestions: This is based on my family's standard hotpot menu:

- Steamboat with dual compartments for 2 different soup flavours: We normally have one spicy soup and one herbal tonic soup. You can brew your own or get the pre-made soup pastes in Asian stores. We like the

Chongqing style soup pastes because that region in China is famous for their hotpot.

- Mushrooms: enoki or button mushrooms
- Greens: baby bok choy, spinach
- Meats: thin cut meat slices (beef, lamb, pork). You can get hotpot ready frozen slices in Asian grocers.
- Seafood: fish ball, fish cake, imitation crab meat
- Quail eggs: hard-boiled and peeled. Just cook briefly in the soup to warm up the egg.
- Noodles at the end!

A CHILDHOOD MEMORY

My mom and dad always cooked noodles in the soup toward the end of a hotpot meal. They said the soup had been further seasoned with lots of flavour after cooking all the other food. My dad would crack a chicken egg in with the noodles and soup and then finish everything in the hotpot!

A Malaysian Sensation

For a more Malaysian experience, you can add the following dishes to your party menu:

Ang ku kueh: *Kueh*, or *kuih*, are steamed dessert cakes from Malaysian Nyonya culture, or the Peranakans. The Peranakans are descendants of Malay-Chinese heritage from back in the Malacca Sultanate days, when an Indonesian prince started his kingdom in Malacca. This dessert is usually served in the shape of a tortoise shell during baby's full-moon and/or 100th day to symbolise longevity. To find recipes online, search using these keywords: *ang ku kueh*, *kuih*, *red tortoise cake*, and *tortoise kueh*.

***Yee Sang* Prosperity Salad Toss**: This is a Chinese New Year tradition that is very unique to the Malaysian Chinese. We gather tightly around a huge round plate of *yee sang* salad and start mixing it together on cue while shouting out our wishes for the new year.

This tradition was started by a Chinese immigrant, Mr. Loke Ching Fatt, after the Japanese occupation of Malaya in the 1940s was over. He modified a mainland Chinese tradition of eating raw fish on the seventh day of Chinese New Year (also known as "all humans birthday") into a colourful, delicious, and fun dish. He was an enterprising man who created this recipe as part of an effort to revive his catering business to support his family after the war.[30]

This salad toss is a very popular, boisterous, and fun activity throughout the Chinese New Year. And since it signifies all the good things and well wishes one could ask for, my mother and I felt this was a wholesome tradition to borrow for a baby's 100th day celebration when there's more people to partake in this activity. We also really love eating this dish and any excuse for a loud gathering of shouting well wishes over delicious food is reason enough!

See the appendix of this book for my recipe for the *Yee Sang* Prosperity Salad and instructions for celebrating the salad toss.

---

30. "Singapore Didn't Invent *Cny Yee Sang*, This Seremban Man Did!" Cilisos, last modified 13 February, 2021, https://cilisos.my/the-chinese-didnt-invent-cny-yee-sang-this-seremban-man-did.

NOTE FOR PARTNERS, SPOUSES, FAMILY, AND FRIENDS

Traditionally, there are some Chinese gifts you can give to the baby. As a modern twist, I encourage you to also give similar gifts to the new mom. If they don't fancy the traditional gifts below, ask them what their love language is and gift them according to that!

- *Ang pau or hong bao*: Red packets for the baby with money inside. Give auspicious amounts that end with the number 8!
- **Gold and silver accessories:** anklets, bracelets, earrings, necklaces, pendants, rings. It's up to you how fancy you want to get with these gifts.
- **Jade:** Jade stones are very valuable to the Chinese. Jade bracelets and pendants are popular. Green is the most common colour but there are others to choose from. Gift the baby whichever colour speaks to you!

And finally, the best gift is the gift of convenience in our super busy modern lifestyle. Bring some dishes for the party! Help prepare and clean up after. Help organise the parties.

Conclusion

Where "Yin" Meets "Yang"

*Finding Harmony between Modern
and Traditional Postpartum Practices*

My modern confinement philosophy is not here to replace the traditional Chinese confinement experience. It's here to help a traditional custom maintain a space in our modern world. To be relevant to the changing needs of new moms and their families. To give some power back to new moms after so much sacrifice and having no control over the pregnancy and birth. And to bring elders, modern moms, and modern dads together by getting closely involved in this sacred ritual of motherhood.

Building this bridge between modernity and tradition allows us to meet at the centre despite how rough or quiet the waters are beneath our feet.

Most important, a modern confinement practice provides an option to the modern woman who wants to explore motherhood through her heritage. For her to start building bridges within herself as she figures out her new identity and how to honour all parts of herself. Finally, she can confidently pass this wisdom down to her children when the time comes.

Appendix

Recipes

RED DATES GINGER TEA: MY FAVOURITE HOMEMADE TEA

Here's my super simple version using the *agak-agak* method.
(*Agak-Agak* = Estimate)
   Be confident and follow your flavour profile!

Ingredients:

- Peeled ginger cut into chunks
- Whole red dates—rinse them before using: If you want to remove the seed before boiling, soak them overnight in room temperature water till they soften and then remove the seeds.

Method:

- I used a stock pot filled with water on high heat
- Chucked 2 handfuls of peeled ginger chunks in because I like my ginger tea strong
- Threw in a big bag of red dates because I LOVE the flavour

- Once the water boils, lower the heat and simmer for about 2–3 hours
- Serve as is or with your favourite milk
- Save the red dates pulp and boiled ginger. Blend them into a paste to use for other savoury dishes!

Tips:

- You can leave it to simmer a little longer to extract more flavour. I found that simmering for 2.5 hours and then letting it sit for an hour brings out the flavour very nicely.
- Bottle your tea and cool it before freezing. To allow liquid expansion and not break your bottles in the freezer, leave some space at the top and freeze the bottle without the cap on.
- You can top up the pot for a second boil to make teas to last you a week or two.
- Family members can drink this too. It's still tasty when served cold!

YEE SANG PROSPERITY SALAD RECIPE

Special "K" Sauce: Yes, I added things to a sauce recipe my mom gave me to make it my own! Just mix the ingredients below together and adjust the flavour as needed. You guys *agak-agak, lah*! (*agak-agak*: Malay word for "estimate"). Set aside in a bowl.

- 1 cup plum sauce
- ½ Tbsp hoisin sauce
- 3 Tbsp honey

- 3 Tbsp lemon juice (or lime)
- ½ tsp five spice powder
- 1 Tbsp fruit jam (apricot jam is my choice)
- 3 tsp sesame oil
- salt to taste

Salad Components: Preferably, arrange your salad in a large round plate. This can be a cheese platter plate or a big serving plate. In Chinese culture, circles and round shapes signify unity and are an auspicious shape in *feng shui*.

Multicoloured Vegetables: Easiest to get and prepare are spiralised carrots and cucumbers, thinly sliced and blanched red cabbage, and red and yellow capsicums (also known as bell peppers) sliced thinly.

Fruits: Berries are a nice touch for flavour and colour. Mandarin oranges signify gold ingots, so I like using these.

Crunchy components: Get pre-made wanton skins from any Asian grocer, or egg roll skins from a Western grocer. Cut them into pinkie finger–sized rectangles and fry in oil. Remove when lightly browned. You can put these into ziplock bags or in bowls in preparation for the salad toss.

Seasoning: Use spoons or small Asian sauce dishes to separately hold ½ tsp of white pepper, ½ tsp of five spice powder, and 1 Tbsp of roasted sesame seeds.

Fish: Your choice of smoked or raw fish (like sashimi cuts). My family likes smoked salmon.

Instructions

How many veggies should you prepare? Honestly, I've always eyeballed the amount based on how much sauce there is. Once again, *agak-agak, lah!*

Arrange the veggies on the round plate. Alternate different colours. Scatter the fruits on top of the veggies. Place the fish right at the top in the center.

Have chopsticks ready for the toss! It's easier to use chopsticks to mix this salad than forks.

Place the plate in the center of the table where you'll be gathering to perform the toss. Place the other salad components around the plate and snap a picture!

Now, crunch up the fried wanton skins and scatter them around on the salad. Do the same with the seasoning and sauce.

Then gather everyone around the plate and make sure they all have a pair of chopsticks. Place the end of the chopstick at the edge of the plate just touching the salad. Ready?

Have someone count down, "One, two, three . . ." and start the symphony of noise while mixing the salad together!

"HEALTHY BABY AND MOMMY!"

"LUCKY BABY!"

"GOOD LUCK FOR THE FAMILY!"

Remember to toss the salad in a civilised manner so that you have enough to eat! It can get messy, but everyone can also toss the salad calmly to keep as much of it on the plate.

Acknowledgments

This book baby was carried to term—and the author in me was born—thanks to the nurturing of the following individuals and groups:

Ken, my husband and cheerleader. Thank you for being my anchor and grounding me when I'm flying too high in my clouds of ideas, and for being the fire that lifts my hot air balloon through the storm of doubts.

Tracie, thank you for being my daydreaming and brainstorming buddy and for encouraging me to take the many leaps I've been hesitant about.

To the women of my Authors Who Lead book group, Heather, Melissa, and Katt. I miss the six months we've spent growing our books together. I appreciate how we've always felt safe enough with each other to be able to be vulnerable during our group meetings.

Azul, I didn't know how much my life would change when we first had our call. I'm thankful for you as a mentor in my writing journey and in my entrepreneurship adventure. It's been an incredible period of growth.

Dr. Eun Kim, thank you for being equally excited about this book and for generously sharing your expertise and resources of Traditional Chinese Medicine with me.

Ann, I will always remember my first experience with you as the developmental editor. You gave me a much-needed confidence boost that I was heading in the right direction with my writing.

Mandala Tree Press team: Kim, Emily, Kaitlin, Amanda, thank you for carrying me all the way to the finish line.

Amanda and Pey Shyan, my fellow medical colleagues, thank you for answering all my questions about postpartum care and for sharing your personal stories and opinions about our Chinese confinement practice. Thank you for showing me that the modern medical woman can also be deeply in touch with her traditional roots.

Finally, to the Women of the Asian Hustle Network (AHN) and the rest of the AHN Facebook community, I will always remember the stepping stones you guys provided that helped me take the leap of faith to take this book idea to the next level.

About the Author

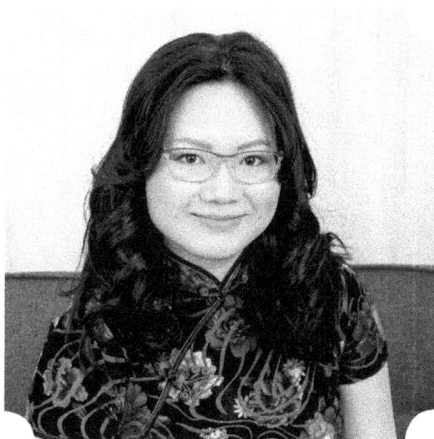

After becoming a physician and practicing medicine in Australia, Dr. Kristal Lau got her MS degree in Public Health. She believes that the future of health lies in combining our past and present knowledge about healing to meet the needs of our constantly evolving society as we move forward.

Kristal grew up in Malaysia, where it's common for people to use modern medicine alongside traditional medicine. She frequently applied this concept when managing her patients and their families—as long as the medical treatments and traditional or home remedies don't clash and cause harm.

After moving away from Australia in 2017, Kristal rebranded herself as a "Physician-turned-Postpartum Wellness Consultant," taking her medical training and practical experience and using that to explore her interests in writing and podcasting. Now, Kristal runs a small business, called Mama's Wing Woman, offering postpartum support to new moms and their growing families.

Kristal and her husband have four children: two cheeky daughters and two incorrigible fur babies. Kristal practiced confinement after her first child with her mom as her confinement person. She's since completed her second confinement practice with her husband as her support person.